4th Edition

Communication & Interpersonal Skills in Nursing

Sara Miller McCune founded SAGE Publishing in 1965 to support the dissemination of usable knowledge and educate a global community. SAGE publishes more than 1000 journals and over 800 new books each year, spanning a wide range of subject areas. Our growing selection of library products includes archives, data, case studies and video. SAGE remains majority owned by our founder and after her lifetime will become owned by a charitable trust that secures the company's continued independence.

Los Angeles | London | New Delhi | Singapore | Washington DC | Melbourne

4ᵗʰ Edition

Communication & Interpersonal Skills in Nursing

Alec Grant &
Benny Goodman

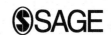

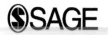

Learning Matters
An imprint of SAGE Publications Ltd
1 Oliver's Yard
55 City Road
London EC1Y 1SP

SAGE Publications Inc.
2455 Teller Road
Thousand Oaks, California 91320

SAGE Publications India Pvt Ltd
B 1/I 1 Mohan Cooperative Industrial Area
Mathura Road
New Delhi 110 044

SAGE Publications Asia-Pacific Pte Ltd
3 Church Street
#10-04 Samsung Hub
Singapore 049483

First edition published 2009 by Learning Matters Ltd
Second edition published 2011
Third edition published 2015
Fourth edition published 2019

Editor: Donna Goddard
Development editor: Richenda Milton-Daws
Senior project editor: Chris Marke
Project management: Swales and Willis Ltd, Exeter, Devon
Marketing manager: Tamara Navaratnam
Cover design: Wendy Scott
Typeset by: C&M Digitals (P) Ltd, Chennai, India
Printed in the UK

Library of Congress Control Number: 2017961768

British Library Cataloguing in Publication data

A catalogue record for this book is available from the British Library

ISBN 978-1-5264-0098-7
ISBN 978-1-5264-0099-4 (pbk)

At SAGE we take sustainability seriously. Most of our products are printed in the UK using responsibly sourced papers and boards. When we print overseas we ensure sustainable papers are used as measured by the PREPS grading system. We undertake an annual audit to monitor our sustainability.

Contents

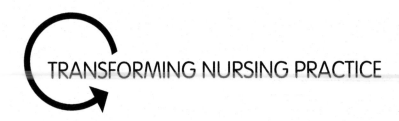

TRANSFORMING NURSING PRACTICE

Transforming Nursing Practice is a series tailor made for pre-registration students nurses. Each book in the series is:

 Affordable

 Full of active learning features

 Mapped to the NMC Standards of proficiency for registered nurses

 Focused on applying theory to practice

Each book addresses a core topic and they have been carefully developed to be simple to use, quick to read and written in clear language.

An invaluable series of books that explicitly relates to the NMC standards. Each book covers a different topic that students need to explore in order to develop into a qualified nurse... I would recommend this series to all Pre-Registered nursing students whatever their field or year of study.

LINDA ROBSON,
Senior Lecturer at Edge Hill University

Many titles in the series are on our recommended reading list and for good reason - the content is up to date and easy to read. These are the books that actually get used beyond training and into your nursing career.

EMMA LYDON,
Adult Student Nursing

ABOUT THE SERIES EDITORS

DR MOOI STANDING is an Independent Nursing Consultant (UK and International) and is responsible for the core knowledge, adult nursing and personal and professional learning skills titles. She is an experienced NMC Quality Assurance Reviewer of educational programmes and a Professional Regulator Panellist on the NMC Practice Committee. Mooi is also Board member of Special Olympics Malaysia, enabling people with intellectual disabilities to participate in sports and athletics nationally and internationally.

DR SANDRA WALKER is a Clinical Academic in Mental Health working between Southern Health Trust and the University of Southampton and responsible for the mental health nursing titles. She is a Qualified Mental Health Nurse with a wide range of clinical experience spanning more than 25 years.

BESTSELLING TEXTBOOKS

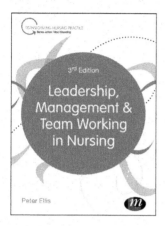

3rd Edition

Leadership, Management & Team Working in Nursing

Peter Ellis

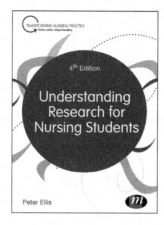

4th Edition

Understanding Research for Nursing Students

Peter Ellis

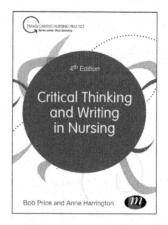

4th Edition

Critical Thinking and Writing in Nursing

Bob Price and Anne Harrington

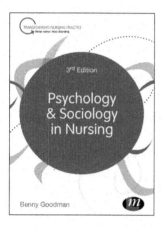

3rd Edition

Psychology & Sociology in Nursing

Benny Goodman

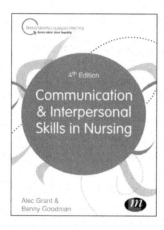

4th Edition

Communication & Interpersonal Skills in Nursing

Alec Grant & Benny Goodman

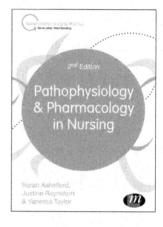

2nd Edition

Pathophysiology & Pharmacology in Nursing

Sarah Ashelford, Justine Raynsford & Vanessa Taylor

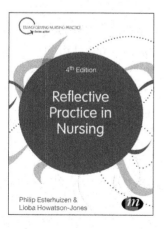

4th Edition

Reflective Practice in Nursing

Philip Esterhuizen & Lioba Howatson-Jones

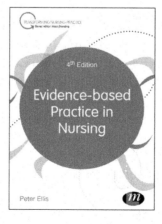

4th Edition

Evidence-based Practice in Nursing

Peter Ellis

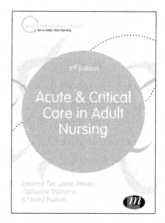

3rd Edition

Acute & Critical Care in Adult Nursing

Desiree Tait, Jane James, Catherine Williams & David Barton

You can find a full list of textbooks in the
Transforming Nursing Practice series at
https://uk.sagepub.com

Foreword by Professor Graham Scambler

Nurse education has developed considerably since the early days of degree courses, and one of its primary resources has been the increasing sophisticated body of theory and research emanating from the social sciences. It is one thing to note this, however, and quite another to find ways of screening, editing and translating this sometimes arcane and conceptually challenging literature into an applied and expedient form for nursing students and practitioners. The authors of the fourth edition of *Communication and Interpersonal Skills* pull off precisely this feat. Moreover they do so in an especially logical, sensitive and compelling manner.

Arguably, the urgency of this task has rarely been greater. At the time of writing we are well into a fourth decade of 'financial' capitalism, or 'neoliberalism', which has culminated in a sustained attack on the post-war welfare state. The nursing profession, long at the sharp end of delivering treatment and care, has found itself coping under considerable collective and personal strain. While it would be foolish to suggest that this strain can be dissipated by a textbook, however appealing, it is I think reasonable to argue that critical thinking and a fully contextualised understanding of contemporary nursing practice can be (a) genuine counters to demoralisation and (b) triggers for positive engagement.

The text invites readers to follow a sequence of steps from understanding professional statements on the importance of communication and interpersonal skills (CIPS) to understanding the implications of CIPS for good practice in twenty-first century nursing. The text is so designed as to coax its readers step by step towards a comprehensive grasp of CIPS in practice. The authors start by introducing a series of salient concepts, and do so in a way that makes them accessible to neophyte readers. This is followed by a consideration of evidence and the importance of a credible and comprehensive evidence base for nursing, stretching from the biological to the social, cultural and environmental. A discussion of the functions of CIPS and barriers to their effectiveness is succeeded by an illustrated discourse on the integration of theory and practice in nursing. The broader environmental frame within which all nursing is necessarily undertaken is addressed next, followed by examinations of cultural diversity and the moral issues that arise across all fields of nursing practice. Attention is given to the concept of reflexivity, or the capacity for self-interrogation, with reference to CIPS. Nursing, the authors insist (rightly in my view), is not just a matter of nurse–patient relations. It is not solely an issue of professional competence and one-to-one dealings with people who are ill. Every individual encounter takes place in a context shaped by social factors. How is health determined? How are healthcare systems shaped, and to what effect? What role do nurses play in either reproducing the status quo or changing it?

It is still unusual for nurses, doctors and allied health workers to be confronted with, and invited to think through, what it is that they do day-to-day, *not only clinically but as producers, reproducers and potential transformers of the status quo*. Individual nurses may feel powerless to change things, but when they act in concert their voices are far more powerful. Like it or not, nursing has this political dimension; and this is particularly conspicuous post-2010 in general, and in the wake of the 2012 Health and Social Care Act in particular. The National Health Service is undergoing radical 'reform'. I commend this impressive book-cum-manual because it not only underlines basic and vital nursing skills, but also offers students and practitioners the tools to ask of themselves just what it is that they are doing for those they serve and how it might be done better. Nurses should and must comprise an active citizenry; they are no longer passive purveyors of semi-specialised skill-sets.

Graham Scambler, PhD, FAcSS

Emeritus Professor of Sociology

University College London

Visiting Professor of Sociology

Surrey University

Foreword by Professor Gary Rolfe

Why, we might ask, do we need a book about communication and interpersonal skills (CIPS) written specifically for nurses? The answer is both simple and complex. The simple answer is that nursing is an interpersonal practice that has a special concern with clear and effective communication. We might almost say that nursing *is* a special form of communicating, which is sometimes referred to as the 'therapeutic relationship'. The more complex answer, which is addressed in great detail in this book, is that communication is not simply a technique to be applied or administered *by* the nurse *to* the patient. Nor are the skills involved in interpersonal communication to be compared with the skill of, say, making a bed or applying a sterile dressing. That is to say, there is no 'one size fits all' procedure that, if followed rigorously, will result in the perfectly clear and unambiguous communication of a thought or idea in the nurse's head directly to the head of the patient.

The philosopher Ludwig Wittgenstein suggested that communication, whether spoken, written or conveyed non-verbally, was not a simple and transparent interaction, and that 'telling' was far more complex than we might first imagine. He asks:

> But how is **telling** done? When are we said to **tell** anything? What is the language game of telling? I should like to say: you regard it as much too much a matter of course that one can tell anything to anyone. That is to say: we are so much accustomed to communication through language, in conversation, that it looks to us as if the whole point of communication lay in this: someone else grasps the sense of my words – which is something mental: he as it were takes it into his own mind.
>
> (Wittgenstein, 1972, p114)

This is the very point that Grant and Goodman make in the Introduction to this volume: it is always dangerous to take our ability to communicate for granted; to assume that when we tell something to another person we are performing a kind of telepathy in which a thought or idea is transmitted more or less accurately from one mind to another. And we should not forget that lines of communication flow in both directions and that, for the nurse, the ability to tell or instruct the patient is only half the story, and perhaps not even the most important half. The nurse must also be open to hear and understand what the patient is saying, and that is no easy task since patients in mental and physical distress often convey their messages through metaphor, through simile, and sometimes through their physical actions or other non-verbal means.

Communication, then, is not just concerned with straightforward telling or instructing – it is a complex social process in which both parties come to an agreement about meaning. As Grant and Goodman demonstrate, it cannot be assumed that even a simple message such as asking a patient to take a shower will be accurately heard and clearly understood. Similarly, when a patient tries to communicate the nature and extent of their pain, the nurse must listen, look, interpret and arrive at an agreed understanding. This also applies to communications between the nurse and other members of the multi-disciplinary team. Nurses and doctors often employ what Wittgenstein called different 'language games'. Doctors typically communicate in the language of technical interventions and medical cure, whereas nurses often prefer to talk of therapeutic partnerships and nursing care. At best, this can lead to misunderstanding between team members, and at worse it can result in nurses compromising their beliefs and values in an attempt to communicate with other professions using terms and concepts that are foreign to the practice of nursing.

It therefore bears constant repeating that CIPS is a complex and multi-faceted social activity that needs to be learnt, understood and constantly practised. Hence the urgent need for this book. Communication is a large and important part of what nursing is and what nurses do, and this book fulfils admirably its remit of providing a thorough evidence-based overview of how nurses and patients relate to one another, focusing on both inter- and intra-personal theories and frameworks. However, it does much more. As we have seen, effective communication demands a thorough understanding of the social context in which it occurs, and the latest edition of this book extends its reach in a timely way beyond the individual and beyond the setting in which nursing takes place to a wider discussion of culture, the environment and politics from a critical theory perspective.

Gary Rolfe, PhD

Emeritus Professor of Nursing

Swansea University

About the authors

Alec Grant, PhD is now an independent scholar, having retired from his position as Reader in Narrative Mental Health in the School of Health Sciences at the University of Brighton in May 2017. He qualified as a mental health nurse in the mid-1970s and went on to study psychology, social science and psychotherapy. He is widely published in the fields of ethnography, autoethnography, narrative inquiry, clinical supervision, cognitive behavioural psychotherapy, and communication and interpersonal skills. His current and developing narrative inquiry work draws on poststructural, new materialist and posthuman scholarship.

Benny Goodman is now an independent scholar having retired from his position as Lecturer in Adult Nursing in the School of Nursing and Midwifery at Plymouth University. He qualified as a Registered General Nurse in the 1980s following graduation with a BSc Sociology and Politics. He writes on topics such as sustainability, climate change and health but always within a socio-political framework. He is author and co-author of two other Learning Matters books: *Nursing and Collaborative Practice* and *Psychology and Sociology in Nursing*. Current interests include the socio-political role of the nurse.

Acknowledgements

The authors would like to thank the following University of Brighton students: Kate Morris, Amy Barlow and Jaime Naish for making such helpful suggestions for revisions to the first and second editions of this book. We would also like to thank Emma Lydon and Felicity Allman from the University of Plymouth for their equivalent contributions to this edition. We are grateful to Dr Helen Leigh-Phippard, mental health service user and carer representative, teacher and scholar, for her overview of the third edition and for her helpful comments made from a patient and public involvement perspective. Drs Nina Dunne and Chris Cocking made an invaluable contribution in their respective contributions to Chapter 6 in both the third and fourth editions of this text, on communication and interpersonal skills needed for nurses working with young children, and adolescents and teenagers. Finally, we would like to thank Alex Clabburn, our editor at SAGE, for his support and help across several editions of this book.

We would also like to thank the following for permission to reproduce copyright material:

Arnold, E and Boggs, KU, *Interpersonal Relationships: Professional communication skills for nurses*. Adapted Table 4.1 (p64), 'Comparison of social and professional relationships.' Copyright © 2006, Elsevier, London. Reproduced with kind permission of the publishers.

Hargie, O and Dickson, D, *Skilled Interpersonal Communication: Research, theory and practice*. Copyright © 2004, Routledge, London and New York. Adapted types of self box, p70. Reproduced with kind permission of the publishers.

Narayansamy, A, The ACCESS model: a transcultural nursing practice framework (p134). *British Journal of Nursing*, 11(9): 643–650. Copyright © 2002. Material reproduced with kind permission of the *British Journal of Nursing*.

Rose, D and Pevalin, DJ, 'Social class based on occupation' (pp135–136), 'Classification by socioeconomic group' (pp136–137), 'Operative categories of the National Statistics socio-economic classification (NS-SEC)' (pp137–138), all adapted from *The National Statistics Socio-economic Classification: Origins, development and use*. Institute for Social and Economic Research, University of Essex. Basingstoke: Palgrave Macmillan. Reproduced with kind permission of the publishers.

Every effort has been made to trace all copyright holders within the book, but if any have been inadvertently overlooked, the publisher will be pleased to make the necessary arrangements at the first opportunity.

Introduction

Who is this book for?

This book is primarily intended for degree students of nursing who will inevitably engage with increasingly complex workplace social encounters throughout their course. These encounters will test, hone and, hopefully, gradually improve their *communication and interpersonal skills* (from this point on, the acronym CIPS will be used for convenience). The focus is not on developing knowledge related to any one specific field (Adult, Child, Mental Health or Learning Disabilities), but on supporting development for progress into any field and beyond. This fourth edition refers to the Nursing and Midwifery Council's *Future Nurse: Standards of Proficiency for Registered Nurses* (NMC, 2018) as they pertain to CIPS, although its content is not narrowly defined by these *Standards.* Annexe A of the *Standards* covers communication and relationship management skills. It is relevant to all fields of nursing and is further broken down into four sections:

1. Underpinning communication skills.
2. Communication skills for supporting people to manage their health challenges and prevent ill health.
3. Communication skills for therapeutic intervention.
4. Communication skills for working in professional teams.

Each of these four sections further breaks down into lists of competencies and skills.

The box below contains an extract from Section 1 for your ready reference, but you are advised to access and read the whole document, paying particular attention to this Annexe.

Key section from Annexe A

1. Underpinning communication skills for assessing, planning, providing and managing best practice, evidence-based nursing care

- actively listen, recognise and respond to verbal and non-verbal cues
- use prompts and positive verbal and non-verbal reinforcement

(Continued)

(Continued)

- use appropriate non-verbal communication including touch, eye contact and personal space
- make appropriate use of open and closed questioning
- use caring conversation techniques
- check understanding and use clarification techniques
- be aware of own unconscious bias in communication encounters
- write accurate, clear, legible records and documentation

Why CIPS for nursing?

The fact that we have learned since birth how to express ourselves within our family and friendship groups may lead us to take our ability to communicate for granted. Throughout our lives we have been honing our relationship skills, through trial-and-error or in response to role modelling by influential others. This may result in the assumption that there is no need to think deeply about how we perform these skills. However, although our practice of interpersonal communication has become second nature, there are times when we have experienced interactions that have not gone smoothly. Perhaps we were misunderstood or friends reacted in ways other than expected. We may think that we could have said or done something differently to improve our responses and those of people around us. This indicates that, while we have developed communication skills, we can always learn and improve when it comes to human relationships. There are so many factors influencing how we might behave in various human encounters, especially encounters in our working lives.

Although similar in some respects to everyday social encounters, the interpersonal context of healthcare work places more of a demand on us to take a developing professional attitude to CIPS. The need for sensitive and professionally executed **interpersonal skills** is crucial in the overlapping and frequently shifting contexts of healthcare policy, clinical and care environments, and hierarchies of responsibility, not least in the face of human suffering. This backdrop hopefully indicates that the practice of CIPS for developing healthcare professionals places greater and more complex interpersonal challenges on us than when we communicate or interact with family or friends. This highlights the importance of a professional lifetime learning of increasingly effective communication in healthcare settings, and the related never-ending challenge of learning to become more aware of ourselves and others.

There is ample literature to suggest that healthcare staff do not communicate particularly well in their work settings, failing to accord CIPS the degree of respect it deserves. The fourth edition of this book therefore fulfils an important function. It helps you explore the many factors that impact on communication and relating well to patients, clients, relatives and colleagues, so you may improve your own CIPS.

A word on terminology: the terms 'patient', 'client', 'service user', 'user of …' and 'survivor' will be employed variously, to refer to and describe people engaged in nursing and related healthcare, as contextually appropriate throughout the book. These are not innocent and equivalent words: they each carry different assumptions about the appropriate place of people seeking and receiving help and interventions within healthcare cultures (Speed, 2011). This complexity of terminology has related implications for nurses around the style and function of their interpersonal relationships with the public they serve. For example, the word 'patient' can both denote (describe) and connote (imply) people who are the passive recipients of largely biomedically driven treatment and care. The interpersonal context shifts with the terms 'service user' or 'user' (of services) and 'client'. These terms can signify active participants and consumers in their treatment and care, suggesting a more collaborative and equal relationship between them and nurses within mainstream services.

In contrast, the term 'survivor' is often used by people, mostly in a mental health context, many of whom actively resist aspects of roles of both the passive patient and the active consumer of healthcare. In a sustained critique of what they regard as both biomedical reductionism carried out in the name of 'treatment' and 'care', and abuses perpetrated by institutional psychiatry, 'survivors' frequently locate themselves in opposition to aspects of mainstream health services (Grant and Leigh-Phippard, 2014; Grant et al., 2015a).

The main interpersonal implication emerging from this position is the need for nurses and other healthcare workers to recognise and engage with such people in non-defensive ways. This places a related demand on nurses to engage helpfully in relationships where 'recovery' is framed in personally developmental and existential, rather than medicalised, terms. In those contexts, nurses need to respect the desires of people to develop their lives and identities in ways that are independent, and rejecting, of what they perceive to be control, compliance and abuse agendas in mainstream institutional psychiatric practice (Rapley et al., 2011; Grant and Leigh-Phippard, 2014; Grant et al., 2015a).

Book structure

Chapter 1 introduces the international and national policy and educational context for the nursing practice of CIPS, including *Future Nurse: Standards of Proficiency for Registered Nurses* (NMC, 2018). Against this backdrop, the key concepts of the book are unpacked and defined, and their relevance for student nurses from the first day of training is stressed. Some theoretical communication frameworks are explained, as is the relationship between CIPS and the domains of caring, moral practice, suffering, healthy relating and empathy in nursing.

Chapter 2 covers some key issues in the evidence base underpinning the practice of CIPS in nursing. It begins by summarising the general benefits of the sensitive

practice of CIPS emerging from research on CIPS directly, and from relevant principles emerging from psychotherapy research. The discussion then turns to the historical
development of CIPS research in nursing in the context of evidence-based healthcare.
Evidence-based healthcare is first discussed in conventional terms, where biomedical,
quantitative-experimental research is privileged, then with regard to more contemporary claims about what constitutes 'evidence' from the 'lived experience' paradigm. It
is stressed that the practice of CIPS is inextricably context-bound, always embedded
in time, place, the specific form of the relationship of the communicators and the
organisational frameworks within which communication takes place. Many healthcare environments currently demand briefer forms of CIPS rather than extended
forms drawn from counselling and psychotherapy models. Deriving in large part from
Rogerian therapy, these models are subjected to an extended critique. The discussion
also focuses on the importance of understanding the development and exercise of
schemas and, in related terms, stereotyping and prejudice. The relevance of the concepts of first- and second-level communication is stressed, some of the difficulties in
teaching empathy to nurses are discussed. Finally, organisational threats to the practice
of CIPS in nursing are considered.

Chapter 3 emphasises the importance of the *safe* and *effective* practice of CIPS underpinned by social thinking processes. The chapter explores the many roles you will have
in relation to CIPS, and the core general skills needed in its practice. The phases of
the nurse–patient relationship are discussed in relation to two models. The nature, and
therapeutic potential, of the helping relationship in nursing is examined. Finally, the
patient's role in decision making in the nurse–patient relationship is analysed in relation to recent health policy.

Chapter 4 discusses the factors that act as barriers and impede effective communication
and interpersonal relationships. It begins by investigating the shift you are required to
make in your professional work when moving from social to safe professional relationships and examines the different degrees of intimacy between friend and carer, and
the rules of social engagement. The discussion then turns to the effect that emotions
can have on communication and interpersonal relationships. Other barriers to communication are explored, including how people construct meaning and interpret
communication as a function of this construction. The effect of motivation on communicating health advice is examined. The chapter concludes by considering the nature
of conflict, what causes it and how it can be diffused in healthcare situations.

Chapter 5 helps you begin to engage with your continuing needs for lifelong learning.
Some issues around the integration of theory and practice are explored, in relation to
ways in which learning should be realistic and relevant to your practice and educational
needs. Learning CIPS through experience, or learning by doing, will be emphasised. A
framework for levels of academic qualifications is presented with a discussion on how
this links to practice. The skills deriving from examining this framework will enable you
to operate more effectively within complex care environments for decision making,
and will facilitate problem solving, critical thinking and reflective capacities. Links will

be made with the assessment of practice requirements to enable you to have a clearer idea of how to gain proficiency in skills. The sections on **reflective writing**, learning styles and the characteristics of a skilled performance will help you complete your practice learning assessments in relation to the use of CIPS in your practice learning experiences. Some guidelines are provided for improving communication in relation to some of the different contexts in which you can act as an educator with colleagues and patients. The final section of the chapter looks to your future as a lifelong learner.

Chapter 6 examines the environmental context of CIPS. It begins with a discussion on the importance of CIPS within multidisciplinary team practice and interprofessional working, across different care settings and within safe environments. The chapter then considers the ways in which physical and social-environmental factors shape communication, in relation to working with different populations. In this context, it will be argued that power is utilised to the advantage of some groups and the disadvantage of others. Next, the interrelated concepts of prejudice and schema development (first introduced in Chapter 2) are further explored. The discussion then explores the impact of shifting friendship, family and cultural networks on communication and interpersonal behaviour and skill development. The demands on CIPS arising from British multicultural society are contrasted with institutional racism and its impact on communication in healthcare environments. The chapter ends with a critique of the tendency emerging from humanistic psychology to view CIPS as solely located within the individual. In the light of the preceding argument, it is argued that this 'fallacy of individualism' conveys a naive and overly optimistic picture of human interaction.

Chapter 7 focuses on the interpersonal and ethical contexts of nursing people from different backgrounds and cultures. It begins with a discussion of **immigration** and **migration** to help you understand how diverse ethnic populations in many of our neighbourhoods in the UK have developed. It then explores CIPS in the context of cultural diversity by examining concepts such as cultural preservation, negotiation and repatterning, or restructuring. The need for cultural awareness and cultural competence are examined, and two theories of transcultural care are compared. The discussion then turns to diversity and socio-economic position, in relation to a society that is made up of different groups to which power, influence and opportunities are not always equally granted. The concluding section considers the ethical and moral consequences of communication and personal interactions.

Looking to the future, Chapter 8 helps you situate the practice of CIPS in nursing 'beyond technique' within a set of interlinked professional developmental, cultural, social-organisational, political and moral concerns. You are invited to consider the context of CIPS in critically reflective professional development, where 'technical rationality' is contrasted with 'professional artistry'. We argue that this consideration has implications for social relationships in healthcare practice, and exclusively technical rational approaches to CIPS in nursing practice may trivialise their worth. The sustained practice of critical reflexivity is put forward as a means of helping you remain committed to high-quality CIPS practice and awareness throughout your career.

Chapter 9 is the first of three chapters using critical social science perspectives to think about the wider contextual issues that impact on communication and interpersonal skills. The *macro* structures of CIPs involve the **discourses** used not only to explain what health and illness might be, but also what the appropriate interventions should be. You are invited to consider how understanding and knowledge can be bounded by certain ways of thinking. We particularly focus on dominant ways of knowing which are often taken for granted but which might have detrimental effects on people's experiences.

Chapter 10 invites you to consider your personal growth and self-development, to understand how your sense of self, the way you think, could be related to your action. This applies to other people's actions, some of whom have more powerful ways of speaking (both negative and positive). This chapter focuses on the *micro* structures of CIPs to explore self, one-to-one and small group interaction – all in the wider context outlined in the previous chapter.

Chapter 11 looks at the political structuring and context of CIPS. This acknowledges that political awareness is a key domain of leadership development in nursing and answers long-standing calls for nurses to understand the wider political issues which enable and constrain their daily interactions. It is not concerned with party-political views, nor does it attempt to impose spurious notions of neutrality. As previous chapters argue, the wider context of certain discourses already provide you with a political perspective, whether or not it is acknowledged. We critique the concept of 'neoliberalism' in the context of a literature of health inequalities, management practices and the emerging domain of sustainability, climate change and health. We end by asking you to consider your response.

There is a glossary of key terms at the end of the book. Terms included will appear in **bold** type the first time they are mentioned.

Activities

At various stages within each chapter there are points at which you can break to undertake activities. Undertaking and understanding the activities are important elements of your understanding of the content of each chapter. You are encouraged, where appropriate, to reflect on your practice and consider how the things you have learned from working with patients might inform your understanding of reflection and reflective practice. Other activities will require you to take time away from the book to find out new information that will add to your understanding of the topic under discussion. Some activities challenge you to apply your learning to a question or scenario to help you reflect on issues and practice in more depth. A few activities require you to make observations during your day-to-day life or in the clinical setting. All of these are designed to increase your understanding of the topics under discussion and how they reflect on nursing practice.

Remember, academic study will always require independent work; attending lectures will never be enough to be successful on your programme, and these activities will help to deepen your knowledge and understanding of the issues under scrutiny and give you practice at working on your own.

Chapter 1

Understanding communication and interpersonal skills

Chapter aims

After reading this chapter, you should be able to:

- understand the importance of student nurses making their own assessment of their CIPS, at the start of their pre-registration training programme;
- appreciate the importance of CIPS in relation to national and international nursing policy and educational literature;

- describe communication frameworks governing CIPS;
- understand the relationship between CIPS and caring, moral practice, suffering, self-esteem, empathy, and healthy relating in nursing;
- have an adequate platform from which to develop your knowledge, and related skills, about empathy in CIPS, and its function in humanising nursing care.

Introduction

From very early in the development of humankind, a crucial early skill that emerged and took hold, essential to the survival and development of our species, was the **communication** of ideas. This enabled people to share understandings, protect one another and develop new ways of solving the problems they encountered in their everyday lives to ensure survival. Gradually, they also found ways to express humour, rage, excitement, wonder, fear, desire and jealousy. Different forms of increasingly nuanced communication emerged, including the development of language; methods of language communication in the written and spoken form have continued to evolve over the millennia. Today, we take for granted highly technological methods such as the internet and other electronic formats.

Over the millennia, communication has resulted in the sophisticated development of kinship groups, relationships and myriad forms of social networks. However, although the means of communication have advanced and become more varied and technical, what has not changed is the basic human need to communicate and share ideas.

In this chapter we will begin by emphasising how important it is that you begin to assess your own CIPS, given that you will be expected to use and develop these skills from the start of your nurse preparation programme. We will provide some practical case and clinical scenarios based on what a first-year student may expect to encounter in exercising these skills. We will then explore international and national policy and educational literature pertaining to CIPS, before attempting to unpack and define associated concepts, including the crucial importance of empathy. The chapter will conclude with a discussion on the organisational basis for the practice of CIPS.

The importance of CIPS for student nurses

In Annexe A of *Future Nurse: Standards of Proficiency for Registered Nurses*, the NMC (2018, p27) describes the communication and relationship management skills that are fundamental if professional standards are to be achieved. These skills are necessary for ensuring the safety and safeguarding of people of all ages, their carers and their families.

They also reflect the professional values and expected attitudes and behaviours towards people, their carers and their families.

Right from the start of your nurse education, you are expected to use CIPS to demonstrate that you are able in your practice to ensure the safety of the patients you work with, and their carers and families. You will be expected to demonstrate this within an appropriate set of nursing values, related attitudes and behaviours.

How does this translate into CIPS knowledge and practice? This question will be explored throughout this book. Let us start by considering a single scenario with two different outcomes, demonstrating poor and good practice respectively, in relation to the communication and competency domain for the first progression point criteria. Imagine that you are the student nurse in this scenario.

Scenario: A distressed patient

Jenny is on the first day of her first practice experience in the first year of her nursing education. The only nurse on this particular part of the ward, she notices a small group of relatives gathered around an elderly female patient. The relatives are talking in raised voices and the patient appears distressed by this. Jenny had been asked by the staff nurse on duty to carry out a specific task, involving collecting equipment in another area of the ward. Because she wants to make a good impression on her first day, she wants to carry out this task as quickly as possible so decides to do nothing about the scenario she has just witnessed.

Scenario: Responding to a patient's distress

Susan is on the first day of her first practice experience in the first year of her nursing education. The only nurse on this particular part of the ward, she notices a small group of relatives gathered around an elderly female patient. The relatives are talking in raised voices and the patient appears distressed by this. Susan had been asked by the staff nurse on duty to carry out a specific task, involving collecting equipment in another area of the ward. Although she wants to make a good impression with her new colleagues, she is equally aware of the need to prioritise the care and safety needs of the patient. Despite feeling anxious about her decision and its possible consequences, she interrupts the task she was involved in to report what she has witnessed to the nurse in charge. The nurse in charge responds quickly and tactfully intervenes with the relatives and patient to try to find out what the problem is, in order to facilitate its resolution as quickly as possible.

Consider the differences between the two outcomes of the scenario in relation to the communication and relationship management skills described in Annexe A of the NMC (2018) *Standards*. In the first outcome, Jenny prioritised routine tasks over the need to safeguard the people in her care and their relatives. By choosing this line of action, she failed in her duty to communicate this event properly to the senior nurse on the ward. Finally, by placing her own need to be well thought of over the needs of her patient and relatives, she demonstrated unprofessional values, attitudes and behaviour. In the second outcome, in contrast, Susan properly interrupted the task that was delegated to her in order to communicate what she had witnessed promptly, without going beyond her range of expertise, knowledge and status.

Activity 1.1   Evidence-based practice

Log on to the NMC website (**www.nmc.org.uk**) and enter the title 'Standards of Proficiency for Registered Nurses'. Read through the Introduction and the section 'About these standards'. Then read the whole of Annexe A. How many of these communication and relationship management skills have you had to use in your nursing experience to date?

Hint: This activity will develop your knowledge and awareness of CIPS in relation to your nursing training, and beyond.

International and national policy on CIPS

Reflected in the NMC *Standards for Pre-registration Nursing Education* (2010), the World Health Organization Europe (2003), European Union (2004) and the Department of Health (2010, 2012) have all emphasised the importance of patient-focused communication between health professionals and patients. This is regarded as vital to achieving patient satisfaction, inclusive decision making in caregiving and an efficient health service.

Recent emphasis on dignity and respect from the DH, and professional bodies such as the Royal College of Nursing and NMC, has highlighted the issues for sections of the public that have not received quality care from health professionals. The Dignity in Care Campaign aims to end tolerance of indignity in health and social care services through raising awareness and inspiring people to take action (see useful websites at the end of this chapter). Older people and people with mental health problems and/ or learning disabilities have been highlighted as groups requiring special attention in healthcare services for personalised care. The role of person-centred care and CIPS is integral to the accommodation of these care groups.

In a similar vein, the *Essence of Care* (DH, 2010) was designed to support measures for improving quality, and should contribute to clinical governance at local levels. It helps practitioners and services to take a structured approach to sharing and comparing practice, and with its benchmarks enables them to identify good practice and develop action plans to remedy that which needs improving.

Activity 1.2   Reflection

Recall a care setting you have visited recently and think about the levels of dignity and respect given to the patients or clients in that setting. Would you consider that there needs to be improvement? If yes, identify what you consider wrong with existing levels of dignity and respect given to patients, how you think things should change and the possible barriers to achieving this change.

Hint: This activity will develop your ability to evaluate the practice of CIPS in different healthcare environments, and prepare you for some of the challenges to the practice of effective and skilled CIPS in nursing that you will read about throughout this book.

Key issues from the nursing literature and CIPS

By using an approach that prioritised the needs of the patient in the interaction between nurses and patients or clients, Charlton and colleagues (2008) found that care outcomes were improved in:

- patient satisfaction
- adherence to treatment options
- patient health.

However, there is some evidence to suggest that, while qualified nurses often rate their own communication skills as high, patients report less satisfaction and maintain that communication could be improved. There is also experiential and published evidence that nurses frequently stereotype patient groups, giving them a blanket label as a group, then acting towards each individual in the group as if that label were true.

The teaching of CIPS in nursing education has been criticised for a lack of systematic evaluation and for an unresolved difference between 'the school way' and 'the ward way' (Shields et al., 2012; Stanley et al., 2014). There is thus a need to consider learning these skills in the clinical environment with greater involvement of clinical staff. The aim of this book is therefore to give students an opportunity to think about their own CIPS, and to seek opportunities to work at achieving their CIPS learning outcomes in the practice environment.

Effective communication is essential to both practice and improving interpersonal relationships in the workplace between professional groups and peers. It is generally acknowledged that successful communication is shaped by basic techniques, such as open-ended questions, listening, **empathy** and assertiveness. However, successful interpersonal relationships are also affected by a number of other factors. These include beliefs professionals have about the status and significance of their profession, gender, generation, environmental context and collegiality, and beliefs about cooperation, self-disclosure and reciprocity. These can impede or enhance the outcome of quality communication, depending on how CIPS is understood and defined.

Defining and understanding CIPS

There are many texts written for nurses that seek to explain CIPS. Definitions in the therapeutic communication skills literature and beyond vary from the apparently highly technical and impersonal to the more human, to the contextual meaning of communication in structures of power and social knowledge and practices. Consider the following examples (spanning several decades). Which one(s) appeal to you most, and why?

> *Communication is about the reciprocal process in which messages are sent and received between two or more people.*

> (Balzer-Riley, 2004)

> *Interpersonal communication involves a series of messages or information which people send out to, and receive from, each other through the use of the senses, such as seeing, touching and hearing one another.*

> (Petrie, 1997)

> *Communication is a universal function of humankind, independent of any place, time or context.*

> (Ruesch, 1961)

> *(Discourses as forms of communication are) … ways of constituting knowledge, together with social practices, forms of subjectivity and power relations which inhere in such knowledges and relations between them. Discourses are more than ways of thinking and producing meaning. They constitute the 'nature' of the body, unconscious and conscious mind and emotional life of the subjects they seek to govern.*

> (Weedon, 1987, p

What kinds of factors influenced your choice? Is communication betwee interpersonal communication, simply and only a functional part of life get things done? Or is communication, in addition to its practical pu enriching the quality of our lives as individuals and in groups through skilled inter-personal behaviour? Can communication be used as an instrument of power, to keep ourselves, patients and clients in relatively powerless positions?

The relationship between 'communication' and 'interpersonal skills'

Well-practised communication techniques alone are ineffectual if the central notion of the interpersonal connection goes unacknowledged. In the nursing context, the primary factor is the relationship between nurse and patient or service user, co-worker, relatives or carers. We are unlikely to communicate without some form of relationship, whether through an information leaflet or poster where there is an intention to relate to persons who may or may not be known, or by physically being close to a person in a bed or chair who needs support to prevent suffering, or through a lifesaving intervention or information to prevent further deterioration of a health-related problem.

In this light, Charlton et al. (2008) differentiated between two different communication styles – biomedical and biopsychosocial – in the literature they reviewed. The biomedical style is information-focused, concentrating on specific information on details concerning the patient's condition. The biopsychosocial style, identified as patient-centred communication, has a demonstrable impact on patient outcomes.

Despite policy promoting patient-centred communication, Jones (2007) points out that there is little research in nursing literature discussing interpersonal skills, particularly in nursing education. This is significant in the context of the rich supply of communication skills research and literature more generally. There is also a critique that nursing education is often removed from the realities students experience during their practice learning experiences (Shields et al., 2012), which points to the lack of literature on CIPS in nursing situations in different clinical environments.

Essential trans-environmental communication skills are listening and attending, empathy, information giving and support in the context of a **helping relationship**. The focus needs to be person-centred rather than nurse- or task-focused, and the relationship is a key element. Time spent developing this key relationship is an investment and yet often a precious commodity. Busy wards with high-dependency patients are the norm in many acute care settings, but time spent attempting to understand patients' indi- le (McCabe and Timmins, 2013).

specialty require tailored approaches to CIPS, for example of the dying, or with children, persons with mental health ities or learning difficulties. Equally, different settings, such cy or intensive care, long-stay wards, and clinics and com- mand particular approaches to CIPS. It is the responsibility hat these might be. There is literature and research availa- actice. A good habit to develop is familiarity with literature

08)
people, or
undertaken to
poses, more about

13

searching so that you can find the resources you need to help you with specific settings or care groups. Some of these areas will be covered later in this book, illustrated by case studies. You may be dealing with individuals or groups, for short or long periods of time and in intense emotional situations or circumstances where emotional distance is required. The variety and range of situations are almost infinite.

This discussion so far implies that there are varying forms of interpersonal proximity and degrees of intensity, purpose and significance that make up the interpersonal aspects of communication in nursing. Developing our CIPS effectively in different circumstances and with different people helps us hone our skills, but this must always be done within an ethic of care.

Caring and nursing

Caring is nursing, and nursing is caring.

(Leininger, 1984, p83)

The concept of caring in nursing was a subject of intense interest in the latter decades of the twentieth century (Clarke and Wheeler, 1992; Kyle, 1995). From a perspective that takes into account cultural similarities and differences across individuals and populations, Leininger (1981, 1984) argued that caring in nursing is about the provision of comfort, concern and support, the development of trust and the alleviation of stress. Clearly, whether practised across or within cultures, caring can only be demonstrated when people interact with each other – hence its connection to CIPS.

Interest in conceptualising and defining the concept of caring has developed since the late 1980s. Morse et al. (1991) undertook a detailed analysis of the concept and identified five major areas. These authors saw caring as:

- a human trait
- a moral imperative
- an affect
- an interpersonal interaction
- a therapeutic intervention.

Like Leininger (1984) and Brykczynska (1997), Radsma (1994) considered caring to be an integral component of nursing, although she claimed that nurses have a dilemma in explaining and justifying the significance, meaning and function of nursing care, because they believe it to be so integral to everything that they do. The studies of Benner and Wrubel (1988), Clarke and Wheeler (1992), Lea et al. (1998) and Kitson (2003) are all examples of empirical research identifying the components of caring actions in nursing, and have helped to articulate what the elements of caring are, bringing them into the real world and away from abstract conceptualisation.

Benner et al. (1996) described caring practice in several domains:

- the helping role
- teaching/coaching functions
- diagnostic and patient-monitoring functions
- effective management of rapidly changing situations
- administering and monitoring therapeutic interventions and regimens.

The above conceptualisation of caring is very different from that described in Watson's (1988) transpersonal theory. This theory is organised around concepts such as transpersonalism, phenomenology, the self and the caring occasion, with ten curative factors that guide nursing care. Watson's theory is intended to encompass the whole of nursing; however, it places most emphasis on the experiential, interpersonal processes between the caregiver and recipient. It focuses on caring as a **therapeutic relationship** and attempts to reduce the components of caring to describable parts, so that these parts can be understood and learned. Watson believes that nursing is *a human-to-human relationship in which the person of nurse affects and is affected by the person of the other* (1988, p58). This might usefully be regarded as *relational caring* (Hartrick, 1997). Hartrick suggested that more emphasis should be placed on relationship development than on skills development.

The above conceptualisations lack the political and economic contexts of professional caring. To remedy this, Goodman (2016) suggests that caring is a 'commodity', bought and sold in a market, which in some forms resembles a 'gift' involving reciprocity. However it is an undervalued commodity, manifest in the pay scales experienced by many care workers. This view is reinforced by comments regarding the unaffordability of staffing levels in hospitals (Dunhill and Williams, 2016). This provides the context in which relational or transpersonal caring takes place and which can distort both communication and interpersonal relationships.

Caring in practice

Caring in practice (Spichiger et al., 2005) explores the notion of commitment, and the difference between *technical* care that is embedded in practice and *relational* care that attempts to attune itself to actions engaged with others using experience, perceptiveness and an understanding of the responses of others. These ideas spring from developments and debates in nursing theory about the relationship and embeddedness of caring in nursing.

There have been two main centres for the development of caring science. In the USA this is represented in the work of Jean Watson between the 1970s and 1990s (Watson, 1997). Watson developed pre-existing nursing theory to place caring at the centre of all nursing activities, decisions and practices. In the Scandinavian countries, the work of Katie Erikson (2002) has been pivotal in defining caring science with a more spiritual and ethical approach to caring underpinned by humanistic thinking, concerned with the interests and welfare of humans. This contrasts with the transpersonal and process approaches taken by Watson.

While caring is considered to be a core value in nursing, there are only a handful of education curricula in the UK that have internalised caring into programme structures, although concepts may have been taught in seminars and lectures (Brown, 2011). One reason for this is that, in terms of research driving educational curricula, caring is a tricky and elusive concept to research, requiring qualitative methodologies to do so. Down the years, these methodologies have unfortunately been accorded less worth and status than quantitative-experimental research. Another reason is that caring has been assumed to be an implicit component of nursing practice; that is, until the exposure of exceedingly poor practice in, notably, the Winterbourne View care home (DH, 2012) and NHS Mid Staffordshire Hospital (DH, 2012, 2013; Francis, 2013). This exposure highlighted that these aspects of nursing care are not universally evident in nursing practice. This raises the questions of why the importance of care has not been made more explicit in nurse education curricula.

In a study of caring and culture in the clinical areas, Ousey and Johnson (2007) found that students assumed fundamental and emotional care was the role of health-care workers. The changing boundaries of medical and nursing professional care and responsibilities for care added to this situation. In the work of Maben et al. (2007b), student nurses prior to qualifying expressed high ideals about how they would like to care for patients. They were followed up 4–6, and 11–15 months later once they were qualified. They spoke of those nurses they did not want to emulate, who considered nursing 'just a job' and were not good caring role models. They gave examples of ways they tried to make a difference. Over 70 per cent of these nurses then described how this work was undermined, undervalued and not valued in comparison to task-oriented aspects of the work. Maben and colleagues uncovered a set of covert rules which, together with overwhelming organisational constraints, relentlessly hampered the nursing ideals of the recently qualified. These unwritten rules included hurried physical care, 'don't get involved with patients', 'fit in and don't try to change practice'. This should alert us to the constant danger of potentially caring behaviours becoming less important over time in a student nurse's life as a result of their experiences in practice.

Activity 1.3   Critical thinking

Can you remember an encounter with someone you knew and who you were caring for?

- Describe the components of that encounter from both your own and the other person's perspective.

(Continued)

(Continued)

- Compare this with an encounter with someone you did not know. What differences did you find between the two encounters? For example, what information did you take for granted about both the person you knew and the person you did not know? What was the difference between the two sets of information?

Hint: This activity will help you evaluate the differences between encounters based on personal knowledge of the other and impersonal knowledge. It will also help you in using your imagination to think and feel what it must be like from the other person's perspective – a necessary skill in the development of empathy.

Lifelong learning and CIPS

The NMC *Future Nurse: Standards of Proficiency for Registered Nurses* (2018) stresses that nurses should commit themselves to lifelong learning, to extend the scope of their professional practice safely and effectively and to think in a future-directed and nursing field-related way. This commitment should be made within the full range of, often highly different, multidisciplinary team workplaces. These workplaces should promote safety and responsiveness to the needs of the patients/clients within them.

What would a commitment to these standards mean for the healthcare organisations, and the nurses working in them, that were sensitive to the need for the development of increasingly effective and sophisticated interpersonal communication for nurses and midwives? Writers such as Benner et al. (1996), for example, argue that CIPS are on just as much a continuum from 'novice' to 'expert' as are technical nursing skills. Benner and others (e.g. Frost et al., 2000) assert that highly proficient nurses demonstrate the ability for 'emotional attunement' with their clients. In the context of safe, effective and compassionate organisational work settings, this means that:

Attuned nurses have a capacity to read a situation in a patient and to grasp its emotional tone: to know when something is 'off' when it looks 'ok' on the surface, or to sense that it's actually 'ok' despite appearances to the contrary.

(Frost et al., 2000, p32)

To help improve our CIPS, theorists have explored the manner in which we communicate and relate to one another to provide us with explanations for why and how we carry out what could be considered a fundamental human behaviour. Because so many different factors can affect our ability to communicate, we will be concentrating in the sections that follow on the following crucial aspects: **moral practice, suffering** and **healthy relating**.

Case study: Attunement

Aaliyah, a community nurse visits one of her patients to dress her leg ulcer. She does this on a regular basis and usually finds her patient cheerful and engaging. On this particular day, however, she notices that her patient, although apparently pleasant and cheerful as usual, seems 'off'. Aaliyah doesn't receive any obvious signs to tell her that something is wrong with her patient, but has a 'gut feeling' that something is amiss. She is used to trusting and acting on such instinct, even though she can't rationally articulate its nature or why she trusts it. She spends more time than usual with her patient and, over a cup of tea, sensitively and gently questions her about what might be wrong. The patient discloses that her husband has recently become unwell with suspected heart problems. This has been worrying her since Aaliyah's last visit.

Moral practice

CIPS need to be worked on over the lifespan of a nursing career, within organisations that truly deserve the title of caring. In the facilitation of this, several have, over the years, provided a theoretical foundation that is indispensable. The strands of this foundation illustrate a concern for the ongoing, ethically important development of 'moral' practice (Armstrong, 2006; Clay and Povey, 1983; Wurzbach, 1999). Moral practice amounts to believing that 'good' and 'right' practice is to be desired over practice that is 'bad' and 'wrong'. Moral practice demands we develop sensitivity to the suffering of others.

Suffering

Interpersonal sensitivity, used in the service of helping others within a trusting relation-ship, must be linked to a sensitivity to the suffering of others. From a review of the literature, undertaken to help nurses gain a better conceptual understanding of this area, Rodgers and Cowles (1997) claim that suffering is a complex concept that cannot be readily observed or measured. They argue that suffering's individual and subjective nature means it is experienced uniquely by each individual.

It is equally clear, however, that there are similarities between people who are suffering. First, they show high levels of distress in relation to their physical or mental anguish. Second, suffering individuals give negative meanings to the situations in which they find themselves. These negative meanings may be influenced by the need to guard against the socially stigmatising effects of living with visible or invisible chronic physi-cal conditions or mental health difficulties. In terms of the shared features of suffering, two key words (**loss** and **control**) are particularly important.

According to the authors of the literature examined, the meaning that characterises suffering is quite profound, involving a tremendous sense of the loss of the person's integrity, autonomy, or control over his or her situation or life … In suffering, individuals can be thought of as being in the process of losing their very 'humanity', and all the things that are considered to be related to humanness and dignity.

(Rodgers and Cowles, 1997, p1050)

Activity 1.4   Reflection

Based on your observation of a suffering patient and your own response to this suffering:

- What could be inferred about how the individual experienced suffering?
- On what grounds did you make this inference?
- What communication/interpersonal interventions were helpful/would be helpful/were needed?

Hint: As with the previous activity, this activity will help you in the development of empathy for suffering human beings.

Healthy relating

From the chapter so far, we can make the following summary statements: good CIPS in nursing are respectful, non-exploitative, non-judgemental and not tainted by everyday casualness. They must be based on the careful development of sensitive helping–trusting relationships with individuals who are suffering. This is because of the experiences of loss of control, functions, abilities and other attributes that make such suffering individuals human and provides them with dignity.

However, the above picture of the basis in nursing theory for good, effective and safe CIPS can be further broadened with reference to the NMC *Standards* (2018). The health promotion and education roles of nurses and midwives include a focus that goes beyond a narrow disease orientation to address 'healthy relating'. Healthy relating, in turn, has a developmental basis, a moral basis, a psychological basis and an organisational basis. We will move on to examine each of these now.

The developmental basis for healthy relating

According to Bowlby (1988), relationships between adults mirror the kinds of 'attachment' relationships that can occur between infants and their primary caregivers. In Bowlby's terms, healthy relational living can be described as a series of excursions from a secure base. In **unhealthy relating**, individuals avoid such excursions for fear of abandonment or the removal of their secure base.

There are clear implications emerging from such 'healthy' and 'unhealthy' attachment styles for interpersonal communication between nurses and midwives and their patients or clients. Arguably, the most important of these is that patients may need to be helped to feel reasonably secure in their relationship with nurses. This is achieved through nurses offering their patients/clients time, within which they listen non-judgementally to those they care for. From the perspective of secure relationships, more healthily attached individuals, who feel listened to, understood and supported, will be more able to take risks towards independent living and increased health.

Activity 1.5   Team working

- With your peers, think of children you knew when you were very young. Can you distinguish between those who were timid and shy and those who were very confident 'natural leaders'? How might their respective home and parental environments have contributed to their respective levels of shyness and confidence?
- Think of people you know currently. Can you distinguish between 'non-risk takers' and 'risk takers'? Is there anything about the early lives of each group that may have contributed to their current respective styles around risk?
- Apply the above two scenario questions to yourself, and consider your answers in relation to your own levels of confidence and risk-taking style. Identify people in your family or among your friends who either inhibit or encourage your confidence and risk-taking.
- Now, apply the two scenario questions to patients you know. What kinds of relationships with healthcare staff might help patients feel enabled to take risks towards independent living and increased health?

Hint: This activity will hopefully help you develop greater sensitivity and understanding towards the difficulties patients/clients have in working towards independent living, and your awareness of yourself in this regard.

The moral basis for healthy relating

The provision of time to be listened to (by healthcare professionals) may be a novelty for some people in receipt of nursing care. One reason for this is that they have gone through their lives being treated as objects. This could include being treated as a precious object who must not be damaged in any way, an unwanted object whose presence is a constant nuisance, a useless object who can do nothing right, or a mixture of all these.

The work of the philosopher Martin Buber (1958) is helpful in understanding the ethical basis for healthy relationships. In simplified form, Buber's argument is that we all have a choice to relate to each other either as objects (what he terms 'I–it' relationships) or as full human beings ('I–thou' relationships). Full human relating amounts to the ethical practice of respectful attention to, and respect for, the inner world, feelings, beliefs and viewpoints of the other person.

Using Buber's terminology, the experience of being treated as an 'I' rather than an 'it' is more likely to lead to individuals feeling self-confident and independent, and trusting of their own worth, judgement and feelings. This in turn helps them develop more healthy relationships, both with themselves, in terms of greater **self-esteem**, and with others.

Self-esteem

Self-esteem, or self-worth, can be understood as the emotions resulting from individuals' positive appraisal of their overall effectiveness in the conduct of their lives. Self-esteem is clearly subjective and develops from individuals' perceptions of themselves and their achievements. This is particularly so in interpersonal relationships and relates to the value and significance we place on our view of ourselves – our 'self-concept'.

To complicate matters, a person may have many objective achievements and still have low self-esteem. Conversely, individuals with few achievements who believe they have conducted themselves as well as they could in life can have high self-esteem. In healthcare, patients, clients or service users often experience a lowering of self-esteem because they are unable to function as they would normally. They might previously have had satisfactory levels of self-esteem or an ability to aspire to achieve higher levels.

Yet levels of self-esteem can be maintained throughout periods of ill health if patients are given appropriate levels of support. This works in two ways: either individuals' health creates such a threat to their self-identity that they become emotionally immobilised, or they will be sufficiently challenged by the change in their health that they develop new coping skills resulting in an increase in self-esteem. The nurse's role is to provide support and confirmation of the person's efforts and thus help protect their self-esteem.

The psychological basis for healthy relating

Some individuals who have experienced a lifetime of being mistreated, and who therefore regard themselves in Buber's terms as an 'it', have from a very young age had their inner world of meanings and feelings constantly disregarded by those who have been in the closest contact with them. Those in closest contact with young children are normally their parents and, a little later, their teachers and peers at school. The influence of these close contacts can have a considerable effect on a person's psychological well-being and sense of self-esteem and self-worth. These ideas and interpretations of the meanings of experiences with others form the basis of an individual's own theory of the reasons for things happening the way they do around or to him or her. This is known as the **theory of mind** and plays a large part in influencing the psychological basis for healthy relating to others.

Theory summary: Theory of mind

In a dynamic interactive way, human beings make constant judgements about each other. The 'theory of mind' concept is implicated in social and emotional intelligence (Goleman, 2006; Smith and Grant, 2014) and is linked to the development of compassionate sensibilities (Gilbert, 2009). It refers to how we all make more or less intelligent inferences and guesses about what we think are the causes of each other's behaviours, and what is going through others' minds, based on our levels of neuropsychological development (Baron-Cohen, 2003; Goleman, 2006).

The human ability to have a theory of mind is important for us in order to 'read' and respond to interpersonal situations well enough to get by relatively smoothly, helpfully and with some degree of compassion for others on a day-to-day basis. However, theory of mind is a specific skill and some people vary in their levels of emotional and cognitive attunement with others. At one extreme, individuals described either as psychopathic (Howe, 2013) or as having an antisocial personality disorder (Davidson et al., 2010) have neither the developed abilities for emotional, empathic and cognitive connection with others nor concern about this.

Others experience difficulties in being able to guess what is going on in other people's minds or read their emotions, because of their experience of poor parenting as children. In this group, the fact that their emotions were constantly invalidated by the adults in their lives may result in them having retarded neuropsychological development to the extent that they lack functional compassion for themselves, and thus with others (Arntz and Van Gerderen, 2009; Gilbert, 2009; Grant, 2010b; Howe, 2013). Sometimes, as in the case of how young children are (mis)treated by their parents and/or teachers, it is sadly the case that what's going on in the minds of the former is of little importance to the latter.

The work of Baron-Cohen (2003), although dealing primarily with Asperger's syndrome, has wider implications for the psychological basis of healthy relating (Goleman, 2006). As with the ability to be empathic, described below, people in general differ in their ability to judge accurately the internal world of another, and this truism applies to nurses as much as it does to any other group of people. This has clear implications for the ongoing development of skilled interpersonal communication in nursing. Nursing students should not assume that they are highly skilled in this area, and may have to work hard at developing this ability (Goleman, 2006).

Empathy

Developing empathic sensibilities

The scenario on page 10, of first-year student nurse Jenny's non-response to a patient's distress, illustrates the privileging of what Goffman (1959) described as *impression management* over empathic responding. Impression management refers to the priority given to the need to demonstrate and develop a positive identity in social contexts where we want to enhance our sense of belonging to a specific social group, in line with social identity theory (Tajfel, 1982) and self-categorisation theory (Turner et al., 1987).

In the short term, acting on such a need may provide Jenny with the sense of value, worth and belonging she requires from her qualified nursing colleagues. However, in so doing Jenny is equally making a clear statement about the status of the groups that are *othered* (Canales, 2010). In her case, these are the patients who are supposedly in her 'care' and their relatives, who are, by dint of her actions, treated as having less worth, social status and value compared with her professional reference group. Jenny is also acting as her own role model in replicating longstanding power and communication imbalances, described throughout this text as characteristic of poor interpersonal nursing. She is laying down a template for her own future style of non-responsiveness to patients' interpersonal needs.

Compassionate CIPS requires undergraduate student nurses to behave more like Susan than Jenny, in managing the construction of a social identity which gives equal respect and credence to anti-othering practices and the *humanising* of healthcare as well as the need to be liked and valued by one's colleagues. The need to develop *empathic sensibilities* involves role taking: putting yourself in the place of another person and imagining what it might be like for them to be in that situation. This links to compassionate practice and to the idea from self-categorisation theory that the perception of people as similar to you makes an empathic response from you more likely. This is because you will more readily identify with their pain, on the basis that 'an injury to them is an injury to me' (Levine and Crowther, 2008; Drury et al., 2009). How each student nurse considers the social identity of what it means to be a nurse will influence their actions. For example, Jenny could believe that not interrupting the task she has been given to respond to patient distress corresponds to the nursing social identity she aspires to (that of the task-focused nurse), while Susan sees the social identity of nurses as being *always* about compassion and the unconditional alleviation of distress.

Responding to how patients and clients perceive their life-worlds necessitates the development of empathic sensibilities among nursing students. Developing empathic sensibilities is fundamental to the broader requirement for nursing students to improve on their critical thinking, and requires the increasing honing of the *empathic imagination* life skill. Because the range of possible life-worlds that people occupy is vast in our plural, postmodern and multicultural societies, it's a tall order to expect students and qualified nurses to be empathically geared up to every variant of possible human suffering they may come into contact with. However, you can develop your empathic sensibilities by the regular exercise of empathic imagination. This can be achieved by either engaging with films and books which emphasise the importance of sensitively stepping into the shoes of another, or by reading narratives from people whose lives have been compromised by serious and often tragic interruptions (see Chapter 2).

Activity 1.6   Developing an empathic imagination

Below are two possibilities for honing your empathic imagination:

1.   Check out the fictional psychological profiler, Dr Tony Hill, in the novels of crime writer, Val McDermid (**www.valmcdermid.com**). In these novels, and the television series *Wire in the Blood* which is based on them, McDermid skilfully explores the relationship between Tony Hill with his highly developed empathy skills, and psychopathic criminals, who are grossly deficient in this area. Explore the ways in which Hill's empathic sophistication, and the empathy deficits of the people he helps bring to justice, are related to their respective upbringings. What lessons can you learn from McDermid's work about how you can develop your own empathic imagination?

2.   The *Our Encounters* series of books contains narratives from people who have experienced health-related problems and treatment characterised by poor and unhelpful communication at the hands of health practitioners, including nurses. Try to step into the shoes of these people by reading stories from *Our Encounters with Madness* (Grant et al., 2011), *Our Encounters with Suicide* (Grant et al., 2013), *Our Encounters with Self-Harm* (Baker et al., 2013) or *Our Encounters with Stalking* (Taylor et al., in press). Identify the surprises you experience while reading these stories, and how they made you feel.

Empathy defined

According to Howe (2013), the word 'empathy' entered the English language in the early years of the twentieth century. Its roots are in the Greek word *empatheia*, meaning *to enter feelings from the outside, or to be with a person's feelings, passions or suffering* (Howe, 2013, p9). The capacity to do this is clearly fundamental to understanding, interpreting and compassionately locating meaning in people and their situations, and thus to be successful in human-to-human relating. It is captured succinctly in the shorter definition, provided by Kohut (1984), who described empathy as the capacity to think and feel oneself into the inner life of another person.

From a more specialised psychotherapeutic standpoint, which captures the need for nurses to be able to *demonstrate* empathy to and with the people in their care, Rogers defined empathy as occurring when:

> *the therapist is sensing the feelings and personal meanings which the client is experiencing in each moment, when he [sic] can perceive these from 'inside', as they seem to the client, and when he can successfully communicate something of that understanding to his client.*

> (Rogers, 1967, p62)

Given the importance that theory of mind plays in the psychological basis for healthy relating generally, it seems difficult to argue against the importance for nursing of the ability to enter another person's feelings and, without losing necessary objectivity, see the world through that person's eyes and demonstrate this. However, on the basis of the cumulative evidence from the literature, Lauder et al. (2002) argued that many recipients of healthcare professional interventions, including nursing care, do not believe that professionals understand either their feelings or their perspectives. In addition to constituting a fundamental violation of compassionate interpersonal relating, it is clear that a limited ability to identify with people they care for, or to understand their feelings and perspectives, may lead to substandard care. This will fail to meet the goals and needs of patients and their relatives and/or carers, preventing them from having a collaborative and inclusive role in both problem solving and achieving optimal health outcomes (Sloane, 1993).

Empathy in context

There are two important contexts for the exercise of empathy: the interpersonal context and the organisational context.

The interpersonal context

Greenberg (2007) argued that health workers who display empathy both enable patients and clients to become self-soothing and are more likely to create good emotional relationships with them. The health worker who conveys genuine interest, acceptance, caring, compassion and joy, and no anger, contempt, disgust or fear, creates the environment for a secure emotional bond. On the basis of this argument, nurses' facial, postural and vocal expressions of emotion clearly have the potential to set very different emotional climates. Based on evidence from neuroscience, Greenberg pointed out that patients'/clients' right-brain hemispheres respond more to nurses' facial communication than to nurses' words. Quite simply, patients/clients learn who they are, and how acceptable they are, from the facial expressions of their nurses, irrespective of what nurses actually say to them. Frequently, nurses may 'say the right things' to patients/clients, their relatives and carers, only for their facial expressions to contradict their words, while being completely unaware of the contradiction occurring between the two modes of communication. This results in them appearing at best shallow, patronising and/or insensitive, and at worst downright dishonest.

Case study: Avoiding anger

John is a nursing student in his first year. He was a sensitive, quiet child, one of a large family, in a volatile, sometimes violent, household. He is uncomfortable with patients expressing their anger in his presence, and frequently feels disgust towards such patients. He would far rather avoid such anger, so he begins to act out a pattern of being available only for happy patients. He is not sufficiently aware of this to acknowledge it or to do anything about it. This pattern will go largely unnoticed by qualified staff and will continue after he qualifies as a registered nurse.

In addition to understanding the complexity of an individual's personal theory of mind and its impact on CIPS, being empathic requires the ability not just to think about the mind of the other but to respond to that person's emotional state accurately (Goleman, 2006; Greenberg, 2007). Empathy can therefore be described as the ability to be intuitively aware of what another person is feeling as well as thinking.

Being able to perceive, understand and respond appropriately to another person's emotions is not easy. This is because people can hide or disguise their emotions with behaviours that contradict how they actually feel. We learn how to communicate our understanding of another's feelings through verbal and non-verbal expressions and then (here comes the tricky bit) interpret those signals accurately. In healthcare, this complex interaction takes place in settings that are often far from ideal – for example, on busy wards, being overheard by others, during painful experiences or on hearing bad news.

In these situations, nurses and midwives have to draw upon their professional inner resources to feel the emotions their patient feels, while at the same time maintaining a separate identity. It is important to recognise which feelings belong to the patient and which to the nurse – a difficult skill to learn. Chapter 3 will provide further guidance on developing this ability.

Trust and respect

Other important concepts when judging and engaging with patients in relation to empathy are *trust* and *respect*. Trust is based upon our previous experiences and enables individuals to cope with the world and resolve frustrations about those things that may be unfamiliar or unknown. Respect, in turn contingent on honesty, consistency, faith and hope, is an element of a trusting relationship. Once these elements are established, a sharing of emotions and thoughts can take place.

Empathic attunement

Complementing Benner's views on 'emotional attunement' (see page 18) is Greenberg's (2007) concept of 'empathic attunement' (see also Howe, 2013). Derived from scientific research, empathic attunement suggests that nurses and midwives who convey genuine interest, acceptance and caring are more likely to achieve a secure emotional bond with their patients. In this regard, non-verbal communication is extremely important. Essentially, patients/clients learn how acceptable they are from the facial expressions of healthcare staff.

Case study: Reacting to a patient's story

While sitting by the bedside of one of her patients, a first-year student adult nurse hears a story from the patient's past that makes her feel disturbed and somewhat disgusted. The patient has disclosed that, when she was in her early teens, she had a sexual relationship with her brother, which may or may not have been entirely consensual. Mindful of the importance of facial expression in empathic communication, the nurse makes an effort to match her supportive and sensitive response to the patient's disclosure with a facial expression that signifies care and concern rather than shock and disgust.

What do you think she should say to the patient, and how best should she say it so that her words reasonably cohere with her facial expression, being mindful of the fact that she feels she needs to balance honesty with compassion and non-judgementalism?

The organisational context

The discussion so far has illustrated the importance of nurses and midwives working towards secure rather than insecure attachment styles with their patients/clients, supporting them in a health-promoting way to believe in themselves, and in their emotions and judgements. However, the base for a healthy relationship, and the skilled practice of CIPS, depends in turn upon healthy and health-promoting work settings.

Contemporary nurses need to be able to engage in problem solving, critical thinking and reflection around safe and effective CIPS within the complex and varied care environments that characterise health provision in the twenty-first century. These behaviours should be carried out in the context of multidisciplinary practice, and be fair, professionally and ethically appropriate, as well as responsive to the needs of diverse patient populations.

Environments shape experience

The nature and influence of healthcare organisations is a much neglected area in nursing and health CIPS books. This is surprising, given the strong message emerging from the social psychological literature that organisational social environments play a part in shaping experience and identity (Tajfel, 1982; Turner et al., 1987; Meyerson, 2002; Zimbardo, 2009) at both conscious (rational) and unconscious (including irrational) levels (Morgan, 2006; Alvesson and Spicer, 2012).

Concept summary: External and internal environments

By external environment, we mean all the features that seem external to patients/clients and staff, and that can have an influence on their perception, experience of, reaction to, and involvement in healthcare. These features include inpatient or outpatient healthcare environments, such as wards or clinics, and staff and patient cultures.

Patients' internal environmental state is derived from their physiological, spiritual, psychological, developmental and social characteristics. These internal states will have been influenced by beliefs from family, friends or the media, and by previous experiences of healthcare settings.

Two views of healthcare organisations

Organisational social science suggests that work organisations can be thought about and experienced on a spectrum made up of both irrational and rational features, and that every organisation contains both of these features in different ways (Alvesson and Spicer, 2012). However, at a common-sense level, we often experience the healthcare organisations within which we undertake our practice placements as simply the settings where people work together to carry out the delivery of high-quality nursing care. Positioned squarely in the rational area of the spectrum, this implicit view of organisations suggests that they can be always trusted as constituting reasonable and well-intentioned places to work in. From a rational perspective, the work of the people in the organisation is regarded as separate from the organisation itself or from what people think about the organisation.

However, an entirely different picture of healthcare organisations is possible, sometimes referred to as the 'social constructionist' view of organisations. From a social constructionist perspective, the process of thinking and acting together within specific organisational circumstances contributes over time to a social and cultural agreement about 'the way things are done here'. The socially constructed organisation is simultaneously rational and irrational (Pfeffer, 1981; Grant, 2000; Grant and Townend, 2007; Morgan, 2006; Alvesson and Spicer, 2012).

The social constructionist view of organisations shifts the focus away from naïve 'bricks and mortar' assumptions of what organisations are about. From solely a rational perspective, it could be construed that organisations are simply physical structures within which employees work. In contrast, from a rational and irrational–social constructionist perspective, organisations are social psychological structures that individuals create together in their day-to-day interactions.

When considered in the context of healthcare organisations that function both rationally and irrationally simultaneously, we should not be surprised by the unfortunate fact, reported by many patients/clients and often confirmed by staff, that 'the way things are done' in some work settings is to the disadvantage of the communication and interpersonal needs of patients/clients. This is illustrated in the case study.

Case study: A negative culture

A student nurse is on a practice learning experience in a nursing home that cares for often immobile, elderly clients. He notices that the qualified nurses and assistant nurses often don't speak to their clients as they give them bed baths and feed them. This seems to be part of the 'culture' of the home. Residents are treated as if they are objects rather than human beings, and the nurses seem more interested in their lives outside work. Little or no attention is paid to the esteem needs of the residents who are left to a lonely, monochrome and unstimulating existence rather than a life.

Task versus person orientation

In clear violation of the ethic of healthy relating, in the senses discussed above, patients are frequently treated as objects rather than people. This is because the work culture is task- rather than person-oriented, in spite of, for example, glossy, locally produced mission statements to the contrary, or on the welcoming name boards outside rest homes and nursing homes. According to the seminal research and theorising of Menzies Lyth (1988), nursing task-orientation functions as a social system to defend against anxiety. From this perspective, it is arguably less demanding, or anxiety provoking, to treat patients or clients as 'bodies' to be washed, fed or dressed, rather than as people to be listened to, or to be involved in their care and in healthcare decisions made about them. Menzies Lyth argued that the degree of intimacy that might come with person-oriented care is, at an individual- and organisational-unconscious level, perceived to bring with it the danger of being overwhelmed by sharing in the suffering of patients.

Morgan (2006), another organisational theorist, provides a framework to help us understand the ways in which, at an irrational level, healthcare organisations may unconsciously defend themselves against the guilt that would arise if they honestly admitted that they were task- rather than patient-oriented (see also Chapter 3). Drawing on Freudian principles, Morgan argued that organisations often protect themselves by using *defence mechanisms*. At an individual level, defence mechanisms refer to the ways in which individuals maintain an acceptable social face by defending themselves against blame and guilt, in a way that is outside their awareness. Morgan asserted that this process can occur on a larger scale, at the level of the socially constructed organisation. A common organisational defence mechanism is **rationalisation**. In the context of day-to-day nursing work, rationalisation might be seen to occur when nurses give plausible reasons for not spending time with their clients and listening to their concerns. 'Too busy' or 'not enough time' are often given as rationalised reasons. However, if tasks rather than people denote a deeply engrained work culture, having more time is unlikely to change these cultural practices.

Busyness affecting group and individual behaviour

A 'we're too busy' stance might contain more than a grain of truth in circumstances where there are staff shortages. However, a basic understanding of the ways in which nurses and other healthcare staff think and behave in groups, in relation to how they identify with them at conscious and less than conscious levels, may add to our understanding of the social psychological, organisational processes whereby clients' communication and interpersonal needs are either ignored or treated as an irritant. This may be the case particularly if these needs are seen by staff to conflict with the 'real business' of the healthcare setting.

Patients who seek attention from nursing staff, often for good reasons, may be negatively 'labelled'. This type of mindset, frequently observable in a range of nursing work groups, is defensive and, complementary to Menzies Lyth's and Morgan's theorising, usually serves an anxiety-reduction function. If challenged about this, nurses would be likely to deny any wrongdoing and would probably give a rationalised answer. Mindsets may take the form of 'them and us' thinking, where 'us' is viewed as reasonable and hardworking and 'them' as manipulative and troublesome. Unfortunately, 'them and us' thinking is associated with the production of irrational prejudice (Dixon and Levine, 2012), based on insufficiently informed first impressions, with a failure to read patients/clients correctly and fairly at either empathic or theory-of-mind levels.

Belonging to the group or standing up for patients?

In ending this section, we invite you to engage in a challenge. This is to be aware and to recognise when the healthcare group processes discussed above are happening to the disadvantage of the communication and interpersonal needs of their patients or clients, and to act appropriately. The professional ethics of nursing practice, NMC standards and the need to respond in an emotionally and empathically attuned way to your patient may pull you in one direction, while the need to retain the good opinion of the work group pulls you in the other. At the start of your career, and into the future, how might you resolve this dilemma?

Chapter summary

This chapter has emphasised the importance of making your own assessment of your CIPS at the start of your pre-registration training programme. The role of CIPS has been contextualised in relation to national and international nursing policy and educational literature. Communication frameworks governing CIPS were discussed and analysed, as was the relationship between CIPS and caring, moral practice, suffering, empathy and healthy relating in nursing.

Further reading

Chambers, C and Ryder, E (2009) *Compassion and Caring in Nursing.* Oxford: Radcliffe Publishing.

This book provides a useful, in-depth exploration of the concepts of compassion and caring.

Frost, PJ, Dutton, JE, Worlen, MC and Wilson, A (2000) Narratives of compassion in organizations. In: Fineman, S (ed.) *Emotion in Organizations*, 2nd edn. London: Sage.

Gilbert, P (2009) *The Compassionate Mind.* London: Constable.

Howe, D (2013) *Empathy: What it is and why it matters.* Basingstoke: Palgrave Macmillan.

These three texts provide an evidence-based approach to the development of compassion, and empathy as an integral dimension of compassion. They will help your understanding of how nursing and healthcare can and should be made more human, as an antidote to cold, heartless and unpleasant healthcare environments.

Drury, J, Cocking, C and Reicher, S (2009) Everyone for themselves? A comparative study of crowd solidarity among emergency survivors. *British Journal of Social Psychology*, 48: 487–506.

Levine, M and Crowther, S (2008) The responsive bystander: how social group membership and group size can encourage as well as inhibit bystander intervention. *Journal of Personality and Social Psychology*, 95(6): 1429–1439.

Tajfel, H (ed.) (1982) *Social Identity Intergroup Relations* (pp15–40). Cambridge: Cambridge University Press.

Turner, JC, Hogg, MA, Oakes, PJ, Reicher, SD and Weatherell, MS (1987) *Rediscovering the Social Group: A social categorisation theory.* Oxford: Blackwell.

This collection of books and articles will help you develop your understanding of the relationship between nursing identity, group membership and responsive action.

Useful websites

www.bbcprisonstudy.org

Two UK social psychologists recreated the Stanford prison experiment for a BBC documentary in 2002. This interactive website explores their findings and the implications for the psychology of groups and how we view power, obedience and resistance.

www.compassionatemind.co.uk

Set up in 2006, The Compassionate Mind Foundation aims to promote wellbeing through the scientific understanding and application of compassion. We're sure you will enjoy using this excellent website.

www.dignityincare.org.uk

The website for the Dignity in Care network, which aims to end tolerance of indignity in health and social care services by raising awareness and inspiring people to take action.

www.gov.uk/government/uploads/system/uploads/attachment_data/file/216695/dh_119973. pdf

The Department of Health's Essence of Care series, giving useful guidelines and audit tools that can be downloaded.

Chapter 2 Evidence-based communication and interpersonal skills

Chapter aims

After reading this chapter, you should be able to:

- outline the evidence base for CIPS in nursing;
- understand the differences and tensions between narrow and broad readings of 'evidence-based practice';
- understand key issues in the historical development of research in CIPS in nursing;
- understand the relative contribution of counselling and psychotherapy models for the practice of CIPS;
- understand what is meant by patient first- and second-level forms of communication;
- describe some evidence-based principles for the practice of CIPS.

Introduction

This chapter will enable you to analyse and critically evaluate the literature on evidence-based CIPS relevant to nursing practice. First, we address the question: do CIPS in nursing make a difference? We then explore the significance of CIPS in the NMC *Standards of Proficiency for Registered Nurses*, in relation to both evidence-based nursing practice and evidence-based healthcare, from the perspective of narrow and broader readings of what constitutes the evidence base. Following this, the chapter takes a more focused view of the history and development of research in interpersonal communication in nursing.

The discussion then turns to issues around teaching and learning, and the uptake of skilled interpersonal communication among nurses. You will see that the nursing literature in this area ignores key research and theoretical work on the importance of the context of interpersonal communication, including the organisational, or work-setting, context. From this basis, you will be able to evaluate the relative contribution of counselling and psychotherapy models of CIPS. We argue that, while these models provide useful principles for practice, they must be modified according to work-setting contexts. Their usefulness must also be evaluated in the context of contemporary critiques of the humanistic basis for counselling models popular in nursing and theory and research in social cognition – the study of how people process social information (there is more on social cognition, or social thinking, in Chapter 3). The chapter will end by providing you with a set of evidence-based principles for practice.

Do CIPS make a difference?

Backing up ordinary human experience or common sense, both CIPS research (Hargie, 2011) and, in a complementary way, psychotherapy research (Norcross, 2011) suggest that there is every reason to accept the skilful practice of CIPS makes a positive, healing difference to health service users and their significant others. Specifically, this includes their:

- feeling listened to
- feeling that their concerns are being validated and not trivialised
- feeling supported
- feeling understood.

Evidence-based CIPS in nursing practice

The NMC *Future Nurse: Standards of Proficiency for Registered Nurses* (2018) argues that nursing practice, integrated with theory, needs to be evidence-based, and thus safe. There are good reasons why the safe and effective practice of CIPS in nursing should aim to be evidence-based. With regard to a conventional reading of the meaning of evidence-based nursing, practices are considered safe and effective either because of a developing body of research-based scientific (sometimes called 'empirical') knowledge to support them, or because of theoretical consensus. 'Theoretical consensus' means large-scale agreement, built up over a long time, by communities of nursing practitioners and academics, and scholars from outside the discipline whose work has been seen to have relevance for nursing.

Together, researchers and theorists have contributed to the systematic refinement of nursing CIPS practice. This contrasts strongly with the frequently observed phenomenon of simply relating to, and communicating with, patients/clients in particular styles because 'it's always been done that way' or because 'it's quick and easy'. This also points to CIPS in nursing with people having healthcare needs as being distinct from everyday communication between people in general.

The theory summary introduces you to key fundamental issues and tensions around both the meaning and principles of evidence-based healthcare practice, and the activities and sections that follow it will help you begin to engage with some systematically developed theoretical and scientific concerns.

Evidence-based healthcare from a broader perspective

While acknowledging the worth and obvious benefits of this model of evidence-base, there has been a growing critique of its assumptions, principles and related practices as the *sole* basis for understanding the meaning, practice and extent of evidence-based healthcare. This is because of the argument that the conventional model exclusively derives from and reinforces biomedical understandings of both 'health' and 'recovery', suppresses other forms of understandings, and fails to live up to its claims of neutrality and objectivity (Zeeman et al., 2014a, b).

Theory summary: Evidence-based healthcare from a conventional or narrow perspective

Conventional, or hitherto relatively uncontested understandings, of evidence-based healthcare privileges quantitative-experimental research that demonstrates statistically significant, proven outcomes of experiments. These experiments systematically test out interventions for health problems against control group interventions, to see if the former actually result in health benefits. To strengthen confidence in the results of individual experiments that demonstrate such benefits, systematic reviews of groups of these are then subjected to statistical analysis. This further increases confidence in specific interventions over others. However, research alone is not the only factor in judging the worth of evidence from a conventional perspective. The work of Muir Gray (1997), Trinder and Reynolds (2000) and Sackett et al. (2004) is seminal in representing the view that healthcare practice should be based on the combination of three factors, namely:

- the best available evidence
- the values of society
- the resources available.

These authors argue that the practice of evidence-based healthcare based on conventional understandings of its meaning should be conducted on the basis of an established hierarchy of strength of evidence, described below, where 1 is assumed to be the source of evidence in which healthcare practitioners can have most confidence.

1. Strong evidence from at least one systematic review of multiple and well-designed randomised control trials.
2. Strong evidence from at least one properly designed randomised control trial of an appropriate size.
3. Evidence from well-designed research trials that do not contain randomisation, for example single-group, pre-post, cohort, time series or matched case-control studies.
4. Evidence from well-designed, non-experimental studies from more than one centre or research group.
5. Opinions of respected authorities, based on clinical evidence, descriptive studies, reports or expert committees.

Alternative forms of knowledge, such as service user and practitioner narratives, sometimes described as knowledge from the 'lived experience' paradigm (world-view), yield equally valid but different types of information (e.g. Grant et al., 2011, 2013; Baker, 2013; Grant, 2014a; Grant and Leigh-Phippard, 2014; Grant et al., 2015a). While randomised control trials tell us important things about *outcomes* of experiments on various interventions in health research, they are less concerned with the various ways in which patients and clients *experience* such interventions. To be concerned only with the former at the expense of the latter gives an incomplete, one-dimensional picture of evidence-based healthcare and what it can offer.

For example, with great relevance for CIPS in nursing and healthcare more generally, Charon (2006) and Corbally and Grant (2016) have argued that *narrative competence, or the competence that human beings use to absorb, interpret, and respond to stories,* facilitates empathic, professional and trustworthy practice. In a complementary way, Greenhalgh and Hurwitz (1999) asserted that attention to patients' narratives facilitates methods for addressing existential qualities such as inner hurt, despair, hope, grief and moral pain, which both frequently accompany, and sometimes constitute, the health problems that people experience. Charon, Corbally and Grant, and Greenhalgh and Hurwitz all contend that attention to service users' narratives (stories) of their illnesses provides a framework for approaching their problems holistically and for identifying diagnostic and therapeutic options in more sensitive and nuanced ways. *Writing for Recovery*, for example, is a therapeutic framework for helping people enhance their mental health recovery through engaging in creative writing about their experiences (Taylor et al., 2014).

Activity 2.1   Team working

The meaning of evidence-based healthcare in practice

With a group of fellow students, identify the possible ways in which qualified nurses and other healthcare practitioners might respond to a group discussion of the two different readings of evidence-based healthcare outlined above.

Hint: This activity will prepare you for being able to engage intelligently and in an informed way with future discussions in practice.

You will find possible answers to this activity at the end of the chapter.

The historical development of research in CIPS in nursing

The historical development of an evidence-based interest in CIPS in nursing is well-documented. According to MacLeod Clark (1985), research interest in the area developed throughout the latter half of the twentieth century and included patient satisfaction surveys; studies exploring the benefits of improved communication; observational studies that described and analysed the ways in which nurses and their patients/clients interacted; and studies on the effectiveness of interpersonal skills teaching.

Banister and Kagan (1985) argued that research work on interpersonal skills in nursing was influenced by research traditions in other fields, including sociology, counselling, and social, clinical and management psychology. From these disciplines, a set of desirable skills emerged, particularly social skills, empathy and assertiveness.

Thus, during the latter decades of the twentieth century, nursing interpersonal research was greatly influenced by social skills and assertion training (Davidson, 1985). It was assumed that, in order to develop and hone interpersonal skills, nurses and their patients/clients needed to be both socially skilled and assertive. This was reflected in the circular view that the interpersonally skilled nurse had, by definition, social, assertiveness, and group facilitation skills (Morrison and Burnard, 1991).

Activity 2.2   Evidence-based practice and research

With a group of fellow students, consider what the range of challenges might be with regard to implementing evidence-based CIPS in the work settings you've come across in your practice learning experiences.

Hint: This activity will help develop your awareness that the transfer of evidence-based CIPS to organisational practice is not a straightforward matter.

You will find possible answers to this activity at the end of the chapter.

The relationship between research in CIPS and teaching, experiential learning and organisational practice

The above nursing interpersonal research, in turn, influenced assumptions around developing a 'lifelong learning' approach to acquiring interpersonal skills as a feature of professional development and **experiential learning**:

The most obvious methods of monitoring progress in interpersonal skills development [are] … practising the skills involved and … noticing our changing and developing reactions. The practice element often comes with the job. We are involved in interpersonal relationships every day of our professional lives so there is plenty of time for trying out new behaviour. It has to be noted, however, that the decision to try out new interpersonal behaviour must be a conscious one. It is very easy to attend a workshop on counselling skills and to believe that a lot was gained from it. The truth is of course that the workshop will only have been successful if the learning gained in it is transferred to the 'real' situation. There is always a danger of an interpersonal skills workshop being an 'island' in the middle of a busy working life – something that was interesting at the time, but of little practical value.

(Burnard, 1996, p93)

Activity 2.3   Team working

A group of busy nurses go on a communication course and learn the principles of good CIPS. They return to their ward and, after a month, the ward manager wonders why the number of complaints about poor communication hasn't gone down at all. Discuss as a group why this might be.

Brown et al. (2006) critiqued the standpoint that a communication skill, once learned, can be readily transferred from one context to another. In particular, these authors challenged a central assumption displayed by nurse scholars such as Burnard and others. This is that communication skills deriving from counselling models, which by definition depend on dedicated time, can reasonably be transferred to busier contexts where there is very little time available.

Activity 2.4   Reflection

Think about the various contexts within which you try to communicate effectively with your clients. What are the contextual factors that both facilitate and limit good communication?

Hint: Contexts may be personal, interpersonal or environmental.

Much of the writing on CIPS in nursing fails to adequately attend to the ways in which organisational contextual factors may undermine the practice of skilled inter-personal communication. This is interesting when considered in relation to the fact that although skilled interpersonal communication is talked up in nurse edu-cation and literature, its practice in real-life healthcare situations often leaves a lot to be desired (MacLeod Clark, 1985). Brown et al. (2006) argued that this is not surprising, given the clear contextual differences between what is taught and what is practised:

While practitioners may well have absorbed the professional wisdom about the importance of communication in ensuring good outcomes for clients and themselves, they may well continue using timeworn communicative strategies of the kind that lead to complaints, poor outcomes and a sense of alienation between client and practitioner.

(Brown et al., 2006, p4)

Counselling and psychotherapy models of CIPS and their use in nursing

Despite the concern expressed by Brown and colleagues about the limitations of counselling and psychotherapy models for the practice of skilled interpersonal communication, a look through the literature on CIPS relevant to nursing over the last three decades reveals a central assumption about the relevance of classic models of counselling and psychotherapy for nursing practice (see, for example, Burnard, 1996; Brown et al., 2006; McCabe and Timmins, 2006, 2013).

Clearly, counselling and psychotherapy models have contributed greatly and have transformed nursing theory, knowledge and practice from the mid-twentieth century to date. The work of Carl Rogers (1961), for example, has influenced the shift from a task- to a person-centred and holistic view of nursing care, with specific regard to the adoption of Rogers' 'core conditions' approach to human relating (now known as the 'Rogerian' approach). Rogers identified what he claimed were three *necessary and sufficient* conditions for helping someone change effectively through a good therapeutic relationship. These are:

- acceptance or unconditional positive regard by the nurse for the patient
- the nurse's therapeutic genuineness
- empathy.

The Rogerian approach claims its legitimacy on theoretical grounds and on the basis of the respect accorded to it as a therapeutic tradition since the mid-1970s. In marked contrast, cognitive behavioural psychotherapy has always had a robust and impressive empirical evidence base to support its development. It has also brought major benefits to basic and post-basic mental health nursing practice (Grant et al., 2004, 2008, 2010; Grant, 2010a; Corrie et al., 2016). Since the early 1970s, specialist nurse cognitive behavioural psychotherapists have made a major contribution to the developing theory and practice of both mental health nursing generally and cognitive behavioural psychotherapy specifically (Newell and Gournay, 2000; Grant et al., 2004, 2008, 2010).

Cognitive behavioural approaches have increasingly adopted an integrative stance (Gilbert and Leahy, 2007; Grant et al., 2008, 2010). This means that major theoretical and empirical developments from other paradigms are being incorporated into them.

One such empirical development, having theoretical roots in psychoanalytic psychotherapy and clear relevance for nursing practices, is the concept of 'transference'.

Theory summary: Transference

Psychotherapy theories have long suggested that the mental representations an individual holds about significant others may either facilitate or impede an individual's progress towards recovery. Significant others are individuals that we have either loved or loathed in our earlier life. A new person can be experienced and treated as either a friend or foe in a matter of moments, a process that largely occurs unconsciously (see Chapter 3). In support of psychotherapy theories, and in line with contemporary developments in social cognition research, Miranda and Andersen (2007) argued that transference occurs automatically in everyday life, when representations of significant others are triggered. Transference is thus a process by which people re-experience past relationships in their everyday social relationships and interactions.

Mental representations of significant others exist in memory, and such representations can easily be triggered by relevant cues in any context. Our global views about ourselves and about significant others are linked in memory. Concurrent activation occurs: when one is activated, the other is too. Transference includes assumptions about another's presumed feelings about myself and vice versa, and is directly linked to the concepts of schema, prejudice and stereotyping (see later discussion in this chapter and Chapter 6).

Evaluating counselling and psychotherapy models for interpersonal communication in nursing

In spite of their benefits, the relevance of some counselling and psychotherapeutic principles for day-to-day nursing care has been criticised from several perspectives. Nurses are charged with the ability to be able to demonstrate cultural and political awareness of their societal role and related professional behaviours (see Chapters 6, 8, 9, 10 and 11). There are cultural and political concerns about the exclusive relevance of the **humanistic approach** in general. In a comparison of the Rogerian approach with the view of humans as rational (individualistic) economic beings, Howard (2001) argued that Rogerian counsellors naively concentrate on humans as childlike beings who are not influenced or constrained by the realities of the society in which they live. We should thus be wary of a simplistic understanding, appropriation and practice of **Rogerian principles**. If interpersonal communication is practised independently of the contexts that shape such communication, the differences in organisational power and status between communicators, and the wider power structures that govern their lives, are overlooked.

Further specific criticisms of the relevance of Rogers' core conditions, and related concepts, for nursing practice include challenging the following assumptions:

- that the core conditions are indeed both necessary and sufficient;
- that non-judgementalism is indeed possible between people who are communicating;
- that self-awareness and empathic communication are practised successfully.

These assumptions will be scrutinised in turn.

The core conditions: necessary and sufficient?

From an evidence-based psychotherapeutic perspective, it has long been recognised that, while there is agreement that the core conditions are necessary for good psychotherapeutic relationships, they are often not, in and of themselves, sufficient to help clients with mental health difficulties make changes in themselves and in their lives (see, for example, Thwaites and Bennett-Levy, 2007).

Non-judgementalism

A crucial question that must be asked by nurses interested in the use of Rogerian core conditions for enhancing CIPS is: to what extent is the exercise of non-judgementalism relevant and possible in nursing practice? Based on Rogers' condition of acceptance or unconditional positive regard, humanistic practitioners and writers often advocate non-judgementalism. Burnard (1996, p14) urges health professionals to *try suspending judgement on other people until you fully hear what they say. Even then, try to remain non-judgemental! This skill is one of the basic pre-requisites of effective counselling.*

A major problem with this standpoint is that empirical work in social cognition (social thinking) suggests it is impossible for humans to be non-judgemental. It seems necessary, and often helpful, to take 'cognitive shortcut' judgements to make sense of contextual situations and individuals within those (Augoustinos et al., 2014). As we grow up, we develop **schemas** to make sense of our experiences (see Chapter 6). Schemas are mental structures that contain broad expectations and knowledge of the world. These are more or less adaptive in regard to how they prepare us to engage with people and events in our lives, and include general expectations about people, social roles, social events and how to behave in specific situations (Grant, 2010b; Grant et al., 2010; Hargie, 2011).

However, a major problem for nurses interacting with service users is that schema activation is facilitated by constantly potentially faulty, but normal, psychological decision making, known as 'heuristics' (Kahneman, 2011). Two common heuristics are **confirmation bias** and **fundamental attribution error** (Augoustinos et al., 2014). Confirmation bias leads to building a theory about someone that is inaccurate, while fundamental attribution error can support such flawed theory building. It does so by leading the nurse to assume that a patient's behaviour represents what they are like *all* of the time, without taking into account that such behaviour may simply be being triggered by current situational factors.

Activity 2.5   Research and team working

Do a Wikipedia search for 'confirmation bias' and 'fundamental attribution error'. Discuss in groups their relevance for CIPS with people in your care and their relatives, in your branch of nursing.

Take a few minutes to consider whether there are any individuals, or groups of individuals, who you have a prejudice towards. Having identified an individual or a group, consider what sources of information you are using to inform your prejudice. Equally, think about the things you *don't* know about the individual or group.

Theory summary: Schemas

Different types of schema have been identified (Fiske and Taylor, 1991).

- *Self-schemas* have to do with knowledge of ourselves.
- *Event schemas* (or *scripts*) relate to the sequence of events characterising particular, frequently encountered, situations, such as buying an item from a shop, organising a doctor's appointment or arranging a holiday.
- *Role schemas* guide our expectations of how people should behave according to unspoken rules of gender, race, class, power and influence.
- *Causal schemas* enable us to form judgements about the relationship between cause and effect in our material and social environment, and to adopt problem-solving strategies based on these judgements.
- *Person schemas* enable us to make a judgement about the social categories to fit other people into.

It is useful to think of schemas lying dormant, in the sense that we are not always consciously aware of their influence on our emotions, thinking and behaviour. However, there are times when our personal schemas can be activated so that we are more 'in touch' with them (for example, the negatively held self-schema 'I am worthless' may be activated at times of acute stress). Equally, our personally held schemas may be violated (for example, getting into trouble over something when you believe that you've done nothing wrong and that you are a fundamentally good person). The actions of others may also activate the schemas we hold about either other people generally or particular groups of people.

Activity 2.6   Decision making

Imagine that, for the first time in your life, you have been stopped by a policeman who accuses you of speeding while driving. With the different types of schemas in mind, from the theory summary box, consider what schemas about yourself and/or others have been either activated or violated, or both.

Hint: This activity is aimed to help you see the factors at play in schema activation and/or violation. The perspective that we are all at the mercy of our schemas may help you reconsider your previously held beliefs that human beings are simply either 'good' or 'bad'.

In relation to the notion that we should embrace non-judgementalism, it should be clear by now that the human ability to make short-cut judgements has clear advantages and disadvantages. From Activity 2.6, on the one hand, it may be apparent that it is to our advantage to expect what kind of interpersonal encounter is likely to happen in situations where there are clear contextual, situational and relational cues to determine behaviour (Hargie, 2011).

On the other hand, it is equally likely that many of us will make judgements based on prejudice-related stereotyping (Augoustinos et al., 2014). When we stereotype others, we place them in general categories and ignore their individual characteristics. The cost of this is that *we fail to appreciate the complete uniqueness of the whole person, ensuring that our stereotypes sometimes lead us into judgements that are both erroneous and biased* (Tourish, in Long, 1999, p193).

Stereotypes are widely held about social groups and individual people (see also Chapter 6). It is also clear that stereotypes can become self-fulfilling. For example, if a nurse regards all shaven-headed men as potentially aggressive, she or he might act towards them in a defensively belligerent way. This may well precipitate an aggressive reaction from them which, in a circular way, will confirm the nurse's stereotype.

Activity 2.7 Reflection

Take a few minutes to consider whether there are any individuals, or groups of individuals, who you have a prejudice towards. Having identified an individual or a group, consider what sources of information you are using to inform your prejudice. Equally, think about the things you don't know about the individual or group that may have a bearing on you sustaining or dropping your prejudice about them.

Hint: We all develop prejudices as a result of the ways in which we were socialised to life and other people in our early years. Some of us maintain our prejudices by limiting the kinds and sources of information about the world we expose ourselves to – for example, by reading only a particular newspaper, or eating only certain foods.

Case study: Challenging behaviour as communication

Gillian, a first-year student nurse, is sitting in a day room, beside a young woman with learning difficulties. The woman grabs at Gillian's wrist. Gillian feels upset and starts to experience stereotypical thoughts corresponding to a widely held view that clients with learning difficulties are aggressive. The service user continues to pull at Gillian's wrist and starts making screeching noises. After a while, Gillian allows herself to be led by the client, who takes her into the kitchen and towards the tap. Gillian realises that she simply wants a drink. Later, she takes the trouble to find out more about the function of challenging behaviour as a form of communication.

Prejudice and related stereotyping, mediated by confirmation bias and fundamental attribution error, are particularly relevant problems for interpersonal communication in nursing. If, for example, a nurse acts towards a patient 'as if' he or she were completely like the imagined stereotype, and the theory the nurse has quickly developed about him or her, the patient is likely to respond in a defensive or angry way, often because the patient is aware that he or she has been unjustly 'put in a box'. The patient's behaviour may then confirm to the nurse that the prejudiced, stereotyping attitude was 'correct'. The nurse may not be sufficiently aware of the fact that he or she is acting towards the patient on the basis of unfair and inappropriate judgemental attitudes.

Given the inevitability of making instant contextual evaluations about people, and their advantages and disadvantages, it seems reasonable for people to strive towards becoming more constantly and critically aware of the judgements they are making about people rather than trying to be 'non-judgemental' in Burnard's (1996) sense. Critical awareness of such judgements can also, helpfully, contribute to their modification when nurses try to get to know the person behind the stereotype. This requires nurses to practise in a **metacognitive** manner (Hargie, 2011) – in other words, to think about the ways in which they think about other people. Margaret Archer (2003) calls this **'meta reflexivity'** (see Chapter 10).

Self-awareness and empathy

A further question for nurses considering the viability of the humanistic approach for CIPS is: how useful is the concept of **self-awareness** for their practice? It is often argued that self-awareness is a significant tool for improving nurse–patient interaction and should be an integral part of nurse education (e.g. McCabe and Timmins, 2013). It has also been asserted over the years that self-awareness is essential for the successful implementation of the therapeutic relationship, and for the professional and personal development of nurses (Burnard, 1996; McCabe and Timmins, 2013).

It would not be unreasonable to assume it is important to strive towards being as aware as possible of our attitudes and beliefs about others, and our behaviour towards them. However, a fundamental problem with the self-awareness concept is with regard to assumptions of the nature of 'the self' (Holstein and Gubrium, 2000). The notion of the coherent, single and developing self belongs to the philosophical tradition that gave rise to humanistic psychology in the mid-twentieth century, and to related counselling and psychotherapeutic principles and interventions. In line with theoretical and empirical work in contemporary social psychology (Holstein and Gubrium, 2000; Augoustinos et al., 2014) and human and social science (Grant, 2010c, 2013, 2016a, 2016b), it may, however, be more useful to consider ourselves to be often contradictory, multiple selves, rather than coherent and predictable single selves. From this perspective, each one of us is likely to act in different, sometimes surprising and contradictory ways (to both ourselves and others), in different social contexts, thus behaving and experiencing ourselves and others inconsistently over time.

The importance of sensitivity to complex and rapidly changing social contexts, and to the corresponding shifting experiences of self and others, has a crucial implication for nurses who wish to practise safe and effective CIPS that adhere in a balanced way to evidence-based principles. This is that they should try to be constantly mindful of the practice organisational contextual factors within which relationships with patients/clients are embedded, rather than inflexibly trying to adhere to a prescriptive set of communication rules and expectations that assumes context-free and predictable selves.

The organisational climate

Based on a review of the literature, and theoretical and empirical work, Reynolds and Scott (2000) located empathy in the interpersonal context of the healthcare setting.

These authors asserted that patients need to feel safe in their relationships and this depends on the development of trust. Trust in turn depends on the promotion of a culture of warmth and honesty on the part of the nurse, enabling safe disclosure and exploration of the patient's experiences and feelings. This highlights the importance of the evidence-based need to look at the organisational conditions influencing and determining the form and content of interpersonal communication in nursing.

It might then be reasonable to pose the question: what happens when the interpersonal context and climate work against the development and practice of empathy? Supporting the contemporary work on social cognition discussed earlier, in particular the exercise of the five types of schema (self, event, role, causal and person) and stereotyping, Rogers (1961) argued that a barrier to exploration of feelings is a natural tendency to evaluate, disapprove and judge. This seems especially to be the case when a patient's communication is ambiguous or threatening. In these circumstances, nurses can become:

> *defensive, often transmitting this to the client through unwanted advice, failure to respond to direct questions, or curt unfriendly voice tone ... [according to Rogers] ... the logical means of correcting this tendency is to work on achieving genuineness ... once this is established, the work of helping proceeds through the helper's moment-by-moment empathic grasp of the meaning and significance of the client's world.*

> (Reynolds and Scott, 2000, p229)

Research summary: Teaching empathy

Work on enhancing a nurse's ability to be empathic begs two questions: can empathy be taught and, if so, how should it be taught? Richardson et al. (2015) pointed out that the more fundamental question continually dogging this issue is whether empathy, along with the related humanitarian values of caring and compassion, is innate or learnable. These authors argued that the development of empathic awareness and skills can in fact be facilitated among student nurses. They asserted that learning to exploit the therapeutic potential of routine interventions and encounters with patients should be built into nursing curricula as part of a more general framework of 'nursing therapeutics'. In a complementary way, Williams and Stickley (2010) contended that nurse educators have a duty to provide nursing students with an education that engenders empathic understanding. According to them, this can be achieved partly through role modelling such understanding in educators' encounters with students, and through the use of educational interventions that facilitate emotional development. Short and Grant (2016) more recently asserted that such emotional development can be facilitated through embedding poetic inquiry and related arts-based approaches in nursing curricula.

First- and second-level forms of communication

Morse et al. (1992) discussed the differences between nurses behaving in a client/patient-focused or **nurse-focused** way and whether the communication was spontaneous (*first-level*) or learned (*second-level*). According to Morse and colleagues, client/patient-focused, first-level communication is emotionally driven and culturally conditioned, and therefore often an unconscious response on the part of the nurse. This type of communication includes important responses such as pity, sympathy, consolation, compassion, commiseration and reassurance. Often regarded as normal, everyday communication, these responses are undervalued and seen as superficial.

Patient-focused, second-level (learned) communication includes responses such as sharing self, confronting, humour and informative reassurance. This is an important form of communication, but it is vital that the interaction is, relatively speaking, focused more on the client/patient than the nurse (although nurses do have to give some information about themselves).

It should trouble us that nurse-focused, first-level responses include guarding, dehumanising, withdrawing, distancing, labelling and denying, often rationalised within the 'busy nurse' persona (see Chapter 1). Deriving in large part from the work of Menzies Lyth (1988), these can be conscious or unconscious responses that nurses use to detach from difficult or emotionally demanding situations in order to cope with stress or very intense feelings. This results in task- rather than patient-focused work, which tends to isolate patients/clients, making them feel anxious and lonely. Along with task-focused work comes a reduction in good CIPS.

Nurse-focused, second-level communication includes rote or mechanical responses, false pity and false reassurance. Nurses who communicate in this way can appear distant and uncaring to their patients, making patients feel undervalued. This may undermine the trust that they have for nurses and their willingness to talk with nurses about how they are feeling, either physically or psychologically. Second-level communication is characterised by conversation closure statements on the part of the nurses, such as 'don't worry' and 'everything will be fine'. Patients may thus begin to believe that they are over-reacting to their own illnesses. Nurses may, consciously or unconsciously, use this form of communication to prevent patients from verbalising any further fears (Menzies Lyth, 1988). At a conscious level, this may be done because nurses believe they don't have the time to listen. However, at an unconscious level, it may simply signal that the emotions behind their patients' questions are too intense for nurses to deal with.

> ## Case study: 'Fobbing off' a patient
>
> Jack is a first-year student in the mental health field, on a practice learning experience in an acute admission ward. He is approached by Jim, a client in his late 50s, who is concerned about distressing possible side-effects of the new medication he is taking. Jim, clearly scared about what's happening to him physically, has asked Jack several times that morning if his symptoms could be the side-effects of the medication. Jack is aware that the qualified staff are busy on other things, which makes him think that Jim is making an unnecessary fuss over nothing. Because of this, Jack's stock response to Jim is 'Don't worry; everything's going to be fine.' Jim is left frustrated and even more scared. This increases his reassurance-seeking behaviour with Jack, which, in turn, increases Jack's belief that Jim really is a nuisance.

Organisational environmental threats to interpersonal nursing interventions

From an environmental perspective, you can see from the discussion so far that the settings nurses work in often do not lend themselves to the time, consistency and effort required to support patients with CIPS based on counselling or psychotherapeutic interventions. There are two other reasons for this: First, it has long been recognised in the literature of organisational theory that, in spite of realist claims to the contrary by particular organisations (see Chapter 1), their members may be socialised into tacitly held rules of organisations. These rules privilege custom, practice and tradition, and are antagonistic to the uptake and development of either narrow- or broad-reading evidence-based approaches (Pfeffer, 1981; Smircich, 1983; Richardson, 1997; Morgan, 2006; Grant et al., 2015a).

Second, the kind of counselling intervention approaches favoured by advocates of Rogerian principles have been criticised on the grounds of 'naive humanism'. This means that simply trying to create the facilities of empathy, unconditional positive regard and congruence between staff members, and between staff and patients, is unlikely to lead to a desirable level of effective and good CIPS. This is because real or perceived organisational imperatives, such as busyness, lack of time or technical tasks, are likely to get in the way (Brown et al., 2006), and because the implicit, conscious and unconsciously held rules of the organisation governing interpersonal, including staff–patient, relationships, frequently trump practices based on humanistic principles (Menzies Lyth, 1988; Grant et al., 2011; Grant et al., 2015a).

Because of such organisational rules, custom, practice and imperatives, and because of broader trends in contemporary society favouring brief communication, Brown and colleagues argue that an exclusive reliance on counselling and psychotherapy-based communication and interpersonal models have become increasingly old-fashioned.

Blip culture communication

Drawing on the work of Toffler (1980), Brown et al. (2006) argue that we live in a time characterised by **blip culture** forms of interpersonally relating. This means that the leisurely conversations of the past (if such a time ever existed for nurses) were possible only because the organisational context of nursing practice allowed for this. In their view, blip culture health organisational members now only have time for brief interpersonal exchanges with their patients. Although this situation is unfortunate, it poses a clear challenge for nurses to make such brief exchanges as effective and empathic as possible given contextual circumstances.

Implications for nursing practice

The following interrelated set of evidence-based principles for the increasingly skilled practice of interpersonal communication has emerged in this chapter.

- Nurses would do well to consider the limitations of a sole investment in humanistic, counselling models of CIPS. A more empirically sound approach, based on a considered amalgam of narrow and broad readings of EBP, suggests that the person–situation context of communication is crucial.
- Metacognitive practice by nurses (or thinking about how and what they think around their communication with patients) will enable a critically reflexive exploration of their personal thinking styles (see Chapter 8). This may include a focus on self, event, role, causal or person schemas; stereotyping mediated by confirmation bias and fundamental attribution error; unconsciously driven defences against intimacy with patients; and first- and second-level forms of communication. Equally, it may relate to characteristics of the organisational frameworks within which communication takes place.

Turn back to the case study of John (avoiding anger) in Chapter 1. If John is not helped to recognise and change his behaviour, how will it impact on patients, other staff and learners if he rises to the position of charge nurse? Metacognitive practice by nurses is also necessary because of the way they have been socialised into particular organisational communication styles, which may either enhance or threaten skilled interpersonal practice.

Given the principle that all communication is governed by context, although some environments may lend themselves to – albeit unlikely – leisurely interpersonal exchanges, others are inevitably more appropriate for brief, 'blip culture' forms of communication, although great care must be taken to minimise sacrificing contextual depth in brief exchanges. Equally, some organisational contexts may promote ineffective, damaging or abusive types of communication.

From the basis of these principles, it will be useful for nurses to practise the specifics of empathy. This includes empathy both in the interpersonal context and in the work setting, or interpersonal climate, context.

Chapter summary

This chapter has introduced you to key issues in the historical development of research in CIPS in nursing. It has looked at the relationship between research in CIPS and teaching and experiential learning. All communication is governed by context. There are problems in nurses relying solely on humanistic counselling/psychotherapy models of communication. Schema-driven and schema-activated behaviour is relevant to the practice of good CIPS in nursing. Good interpersonal and organisational climates are relevant for the practice of good nursing CIPS.

An understanding of what is meant by patient first- and second-level forms of communication is important. You should be able to demonstrate an appreciation of the organisational environmental threats to counselling and psychotherapy nursing interventions. Finally, you should understand what is meant by 'blip cultures' and the opportunities and constraints for forms of communication emerging from such cultures.

Activities: brief outline answers

Activity 2.1: Team working (p38)

Attitudes may be polarised: some colleagues will diminish or dismiss the value of lived-experience knowledge as being anecdotal, unscientific, ungrateful, 'sob stories', irrelevant; others will describe them as central to understanding good healthcare.

Activity 2.2: Evidence-based practice and research (p39)

Writers such as Schön (1987) and Freshwater and Rolfe (2001) argue that translating research into clinical practice is far from straightforward. These authors maintained this is because of a faulty assumption of *technical rationality* held by those (usually members of research communities) who believe that research outcomes can simply be applied in a straightforward manner in clinical settings. In critiquing this assumption, Schön (1987) uses the metaphor of the high hard ground overlooking a swamp. The high hard ground is the world where research is conducted in a relatively clean, 'sterile' way. The swampland is the messy, murky world of clinical practice where relationships and work are never straightforward and cannot be controlled to the extent that research environments are.

Further reading

Augoustinos, M, Walker, I and Donaghue, N (2014) *Social Cognition: An integrated introduction,* 3rd edn. London: Sage.

This book provides you with contemporary evidence-based information on social cognition, and its relationship with social identity and communication.

Brown, B, Crawford, P and Carter, R (2006) *Evidence-Based Health Communication.* Maidenhead: Open University Press and McGraw-Hill Education.

This book offers a critical evaluation of the kinds of evidence that have been collected concerning both effective communication and the training health professionals receive in communication.

Useful website

http://psychology.wikia.com/wiki/Social_Cognition_Paper_Archive_and_Information_Centre

The website of the Psychology Wiki Social Cognition Paper Archive and Information Center. It gives lots of interesting downloads and links.

Chapter 3 The safe and effective practice of communication and interpersonal skills

NMC Standards of Proficiency for Registered Nurses

This chapter will address the following platforms and proficiencies:

Platform 1: Being an accountable professional

At the point of registration, the registered nurse will be able to:

1.2 Understand and apply relevant legal, regulatory and governance requirements, policies, and ethical frameworks, including any mandatory reporting duties, to all areas of practice, differentiating where appropriate between the devolved legislatures of the United Kingdom.

1.5 Understand the demands of professional practice and demonstrate how to recognise signs of vulnerability in themselves or their colleagues and the action required to minimise risks to health.

Platform 2: Promoting health and preventing ill health

At the point of registration, the registered nurse will be able to:

2.8 Explain and demonstrate the use of up to date approaches to behaviour change to enable people to use their strengths and expertise and make informed choices when managing their own health and making lifestyle adjustments (Annexe A).

Platform 6: Improving safety and quality of care

At the point of registration, the registered nurse will be able to:

6.9 Work with people, their families, carers and colleagues to develop effective improvement strategies for quality and safety, sharing feedback and learning from positive outcomes and experiences, mistakes and adverse outcomes and experiences.

Chapter aims

After reading this chapter, you should be able to:

- understand the importance and relevance of communicating safely and effectively;
- understand the process of social thinking as it pertains to CIPS;
- appreciate the importance of cultural positioning in relation to the practice of CIPS;
- understand the significance of the duration of the nurse–patient relationship and its relevance for the practice of CIPS;
- understand what is meant by the helping relationship in nursing and the role of patients and clients as decision makers in this context.

Introduction

It is generally agreed that CIPS underpin effective and safe relationships. In order to understand the nature of nurse–patient relationships, it is valuable to take time to appreciate the spectrum of those that can occur within nurses' professional lives. The nature of these encounters is as varied as a colour palette, and different nurses in different settings, caring for adults or children, in mental health settings or with clients with learning disabilities, may experience more or less of one particular area of the palette. But, in all likelihood, there will be elements of this palette in all your interpersonal relationships with patients.

Knowing how to respond and react in these many situations can be bewildering if you have to imagine how you will manage these different forms of relationships in order to be effective. This chapter aims to provide a guide in these situations, to help you build your confidence and increase your awareness of yourself in relational contexts. We will explore what it means to be safe and begin by examining some of the theory behind the way we think in social situations and how that influences how we behave. Called **social thinking** processes, these are the covert thought processes by which people process and interpret information from and about themselves and other people. The discussion then turns to the duration of the nurse–patient relationship, the nature of the helping relationship in nursing and how this can have a therapeutic effect. The patient's role in decision making in this context is discussed in relation to recent health policy.

What does 'being safe' mean?

Safety is not the same as risk-aversion. The philosopher Onora O'Neill (2002) argued that we now live in a 'risk' society. The rise of neoliberal politics in the late 1970s in the UK and in other parts of the world (see Chapters 9–11) brought with it a distrust of public sector professionals. This gave rise in turn to audit and other monitoring cultures, resulting, O'Neill argues, in risk-obsessed public services. Patients are risk-assessed, and services are risk-averse for a number of related reasons, including the avoidance of litigation. At worst, this state of affairs can lead to a confusion between reasonable risk reduction and safety. This in turn can result in a perception of patients as constantly risky (for professionals and services) and at risk, all of which can be counter-therapeutic. At a general level, we know that adaptive human development depends on embracing, and risking, the unfamiliar. More specifically, in mental health recovery, the strategy of helping clients engage in behavioural experiments to test out their life-limiting fears encourages acceptable and reasonable risk taking (Grant et al., 2008; Corrie et al., 2016).

'Being safe', in contrast, is a term used to describe how nurse–patient relationships can be conducted without either party being harmed. From the start of your training, you have a duty to provide care safely at all times and people must be able to trust you with their lives and their health. The *Standards* are clear about this – indeed Platform 6 is titled 'Improving Safety and Quality of Care'.

With this in mind, we have to be careful not to cause harm, injury or damage in our communication and interpersonal relationships with patients. Words are powerful, and how people interpret messages from others is where the damage may start. The interpretation of the meanings of words varies from person to person. In addition, we are dealing in healthcare with many words that are unfamiliar to patients until they have understood and learned their meaning. This applies to the names of conditions as well as the phrases and abbreviations we use as short cuts to describe objects, processes, procedures and situations.

The way in which we transmit the words in our messages can be influenced by many factors. Information transmission has to be interpreted and assimilated by both parties in the interaction. Our body language and non-verbal signals can all lead to misunderstanding and confusion if they are not correctly understood by service users and their relatives. This is further complicated by the anxiety patients may have about their health, their previous experiences of healthcare and the relative success of those experiences, their cultural or personalised view of the world and the degree of discomfort or pain they may be experiencing during the communication.

It is not only the interpretation the patient may place on the messages that is important. You, as a nurse, need to interpret patients' responses correctly, so that you know how much they understand about the situation and are sure they have understood what you are saying or are intending to do.

Scenario 1

The pattern goes like this:

1. The student nurse tells the patient that he must have a shower at 6 in preparation for a surgical procedure. The patient is to undergo a routine procedure and has no major health problems.

2. The patient nods, indicating he has understood. The patient has interpreted this as taking a shower at 6 p.m., whereas the student nurse meant 6 a.m. So this is a semi-correct interpretation of the message. The patient is conscious of his health and keeps himself fit and well; however, he is frightened of falling in the shower and does not have a shower at home. At home he has a seat in the bath and uses a shower attachment. The student nurse looks very busy and the patient does not want to be a nuisance, so he does not ask for clarification. The patient is worried about the surgery and has not slept well, so his receptivity of information is compromised by tiredness and anxiety.

3. Because the patient nodded in apparent agreement, the student nurse says something like 'That's OK then' and goes to the next patient.

It's not difficult to anticipate what will happen next. The patient will not have the shower at the correct time. If the student nurse does spot this in time, the patient will take a long time because he is nervous of falling in the shower; he may even fall because he is unaccustomed to using a shower. The surgery is delayed; the operating theatre's schedule is put back, causing inconvenience to patients and staff alike. If the patient were to fall, the surgery would probably be cancelled and the patient would suffer more, in addition to enduring the delayed solution to his original problem.

Let's try it again.

Scenario 2

The pattern goes like this:

1. The student nurse tells the patient that he has to prepare for surgery (this tells the patient what the communication is all about) that morning (this tells the patient when it is going to happen). The patient needs to have a shower at 6 a.m. (It might seem obvious to state the time as this communication is taking place in the morning, but it makes it clearer and reinforces the time frame for the patient.)

(Continued)

(Continued)

2. The student nurse asks the patient if he is comfortable having a shower or is there any other way that he usually has a full wash? (This gives the patient the opportunity to express his personal hygiene methods and confirm that he can shower or describe what he needs to do.)

3. The patient responds by explaining how he usually washes.

4. The student nurse needs to find out not only how, but why, the patient washes in this manner. This can shed light on any fear of falling.

5. The student nurse explores how the facilities on the ward can be adapted to suit the patient and checks whether the patient agrees. As the environment is unfamiliar to the patient and his usual routine is disrupted, it would be additionally helpful if the student nurse were to take the patient to the shower facilities and demonstrate to him how to use the shower.

6. During this encounter, the student nurse can explore with the patient any concerns or anxieties he may have about the preparations for surgery, such as falling in the shower, and at the same time clarify any fears about the surgical procedure if these have not already been elicited during the assessment processes. This takes additional time, but could avoid a great deal of future inconvenience and potential safety issues. It could also provide opportunities to develop the nurse's relationship with the patient and understand his current needs, as well as prepare for their communication postoperatively.

These scenarios illustrate how a simple communication request can involve several aspects of meeting physical and emotional needs. The success of managing these aspects is often due to our abilities to perceive and interpret information. This has been studied in a branch of social psychology termed 'social cognition', or 'social thinking' (Augoustinos et al., 2014), featured in Chapter 2. The aim of social cognition is to find out how people take in information and assimilate it so that it can be used effectively in social and professional encounters.

The process of social thinking

The earlier chapters of this book should have alerted you to the fact that social thinking is the process by which people assimilate and interpret information or thoughts from and about themselves (their intrapersonal world) and other individuals (their interpersonal world). Most of the time our social thinking works well for us. We pay attention to the most, rather than the least, important aspects of our environment, which keeps us safe. We think about people in a way that organises our ideas into categories, so that we can recognise characteristics about people, in a process of social comparison. Comparing what we are encountering with what we have encountered before gives us a frame of reference or benchmark to make judgements. We can also take in all manner of facts, which originate from different sources and experiences, and organise them into categories so that we can recognise them again. Generally, we remember what we need to remember, and make conclusions about facts and ideas, all of which influences how we react and respond in situations.

Finding out more about how social thinking operates is one way to ensure we accurately understand and interpret what people around us are expressing. Our two most common types of reaction to people and events are spontaneous and deliberative. Spontaneous means 'off the top of your head', quick responses, such as 'all experts must be right' or 'all exotic food must taste disgusting'. These quick responses mean that we have not taken the time to gather further information or evidence to verify such judgements.

At other times we engage in more deliberative responses, taking more care to reflect on the event or people's responses. This also gives us the opportunity to break the habitual pattern of spontaneous responding, to delve into things more deeply, and thus arrive at a fuller picture of events, ideas and impressions.

Cognitive stores

Students are often surprised that experienced staff can draw conclusions about complex situations or seem to have an intuitive understanding of patients' needs, without the patients appearing to have directly expressed those needs. One explanation for this is that experienced staff have a store of previous experiences, knowledge of different societal groups and up-to-date knowledge of contemporary research that they synthesise rapidly to form their conclusions. Their spontaneous recipe works for them. However, even the most experienced staff have occasions when they have to further reflect on judgements made on the basis of their cognitive stores to ensure that they are not using habitual stereotypes or outdated research to make their decisions.

Cognitive misers

If staff do not use their cognitive stores effectively, they run the risk of becoming 'cognitive misers' (Augoustinos et al., 2014). Cognitive misers do not put effort into thinking around the problem or situation, and only use the minimum cognitive resources they need. A consequence of this is that some knowledge becomes so automatic that it is incorporated into the organising part of the recipe without any extra effort ever being put into the deliberative stage. Vital information could be overlooked.

Most nurse–patient interactions share features with social interactions more generally, in being dynamic, creative, responsive and socially-constructed and produced. The primary mode of communication is talk enhanced with gestures, personal communication style and body language. This enables all parties in the exchange to share information,

Case study: From spontaneous to deliberative social thinking

Rani is a first-year children's nurse at the start of her morning shift. She passes the bed of Jamie, a five-year-old boy with asthma-related problems. She cheerily waves and says, 'Hiya Jamie, I see your football team won this weekend', and is about to move on when she notices that Jamie looks more serious than usual. She then, momentarily, becomes aware that the kind of greeting that she has given Jamie is part of a start-of-shift ritual that she and other members of staff engage in with all the children in their care, without stopping to focus attention on any one child in particular. Because of this, instead of going on to greet the other children, she sits by Jamie's bed. 'What's up, Jamie? You don't look your usual perky self', she asks. Jamie then discloses that he wants to be a professional footballer when he grows up, but worries that he never will because of his problems. Rani mentally consults her knowledge and research base about recovery from childhood respiratory problems before proceeding to reassure him sensitively but positively.

agree decisions, and develop and maintain the relationship. However, healthcare inter-personal exchanges are often meeting points for a number of different cultures. This frequently results in conflict, where biomedical and other professional cultures don't marry well with the lay cultures of patients (sometimes these cultural positions are described as 'discourses' – see Chapter 9).

The differences between all the cultural areas are around different meanings of 'health', 'illness' and 'recovery', deriving from different sets of perceptions, attitudes, types and sources of knowledge, motivations and agendas. Users' and carers' agen-das will derive from their expectations and experiences of illness, health, consultation and treatments, and sometimes from the re-traumatisation by mental health services that self-identified 'survivors' have experienced (Grant et al., 2015a). In contrast, the agendas of healthcare professionals are likely to reflect their own (usually Western) medical or health-related training together with personal, professional and organisa-tional background factors. Reconciling these differences is one of the major challenges to engaging in a successful nurse–patient relationship.

One simple way to clarify and negotiate through this cultural tension area is to identify two basic goals in nurse–patient interactions: the first goal is associated with information giving and responding to questions, and the second with relationship building. Separating out these goals within interactions can help clarify what will be gained from the interaction. Information giving and responding to question activities are related to enhancing treat-ment compliance and resolving non-compliance, and remembering information, whereas patient satisfaction is related to the socio-emotional aspects of interactions.

For the nurse, there may be a desire for the patient to achieve a satisfactory understand-ing of procedures and processes, whereas the patient may wish to have satisfaction from receiving kindness, empathy, a sense of respect, and being listened to (Corbally and Grant, 2016). Achieving a balance in reaching these respective goals is needed. The responsibility for understanding the balance lies with the nurse, which is why differentiating between the **professional relationship** and the **social relationship** is necessary. This is discussed further in the following chapter.

Case study: Achieving a balance between the two basic goals

Django is a first-year student nurse on a practice learning experience with two community staff nurses, Erica and Chen-Chi. He notices that Erica seems keen to see as many patients as she can in the shortest possible time. Her typical style is to arrive at a patient's home, observe the minimal demands of courtesy before eliciting information from the patient about the problem, provide the appropriate nursing intervention, with instructions, if appropriate, then leave. In contrast, Chen-Chi takes her time and seems to privilege developing empathic and supportive relationships with her patients as an essential part of good community nursing care. Django notices that Chen-Chi's patients reciprocate warmth to her. This contrasts with Erica's patients, who look uncomfortable in her presence.

Roles

We all have multiple roles in life and work, each demanding different – yet often interlinked – identities. Maintaining a social and professional identity as a nurse requires acceptance of this role and an ability to relate to other nurses and healthcare workers. This is not without its difficulties as there are tensions attendant on the role demands of nursing, associated with rank and institutional rituals.

Activity 3.1   Reflection

Think of times when you feel a conflict between your roles as a student and an adult preparing for a professional career and responsibilities. Do some situations evoke conflicting feelings in you – around feeling like a nurse, a parent or a child? How do you manage these conflicting feelings? How does this impact on your relationship with clients or patients? Discuss your responses with other students in a group.

Duration of the nurse–patient relationship

While caution should be exercised about prescriptive rules to guide the formation and the stages of nurse–patient relationships, we can equally accept that there are culture-specific group norms guiding how these relationships should be conducted and the roles within them performed. The rate at which the relationship is formed, and its duration, will vary according to work setting. In a pre-assessment surgical assessment unit you may have only half an hour, whereas on a medical ward a patient may stay for a number of days. Children may have short or long periods of time in hospital. In some mental health environments longer time frames might potentially allow for more in-depth relationships, while community work provides a different pace and context for the stages of relationships to develop in patients' own homes. In residential settings with learning disability clients, relationships have an even longer time span in which to consolidate and develop.

Case study: Ending a relationship

Arya is a first-year student nurse undertaking a practice learning experience in a mental health day care facility.

She has developed a close relationship with Natasha, a young client who is her age. Natasha started attending the facility just after Arya began her practice experience. Natasha was scared at first, but settled in quickly, mainly because Arya took an interest in her and helped her make better sense of the distressing experiences that had led to her referral.

Arya has told Natasha that she is coming to the end of her practice experience and will soon be leaving. Natasha is sad because she regards Arya as her closest friend, and wonders what she will do without her. She is scared to tell Arya this, however, as she worries that Arya might think her silly. Arya has picked up on Natasha's dejection and gently prompts Natasha to voice her feelings and concerns. After listening to Natasha, Arya shares with her that the feelings of fondness are mutual, and also that she believes that their relationship has enabled Natasha to develop confidence in herself that will serve her well in developing future relationships with others. Together, they explore what specific things Natasha might do to achieve this and they also plan to have lunch together to celebrate both their relationship and the significance of its ending.

The helping relationship in nursing

The helping relationship between nurses and people they care for was termed the 'therapeutic relationship' by Henderson (1967, pxx), a seminal nurse theorist. In her terms, this involves *the practice of those nursing activities which have a healing effect or those which result in movement towards health or wellness.*

Theory summary: Human theory of caring

Watson's theory of human caring (Watson, 2015) is useful to consider in this context. It is organised around concepts such as transpersonalism, phenomenology, the self and the caring occasion, with ten curative factors that guide nursing care. The theory is intended to encompass the whole of nursing; however, it places most emphasis on the experiential, interpersonal processes between the caregiver and recipient. It focuses on caring as a therapeutic relationship and attempts to reduce the components of caring to describable parts, so that these parts can be understood and learned. As such, the theory could be criticised for being reductionist. However, reduction of theory to its component parts also enables a complex phenomenon to be better understood. The theory claims to allow for, and be open to, **existential– phenomenological** and spiritual dimensions of caring and healing that cannot be fully explained scientifically through the Western mind of modern society. More information on the theory can be obtained from the web resources found at the end of the chapter.

McMahon's (1993) later, complementary, view was that nursing involves both overt and non-visible caring practices:

- developing the nurse–patient relationship based upon partnership, intimacy and reciprocity;
- manipulating the environment – from the macro (organisational) level, through to the meso (patient environment) level to the micro environment (i.e. the physical features that impact on the wellbeing of the patient);
- teaching – involving patient education and information;
- providing comfort – physical and non-physical care;
- adopting complementary health practices – these are creative approaches to healing that are incorporated into nursing care;
- utilising tested physical interventions – incorporating intuitive approaches to care that can be supported by inductive research approaches.

To help nurses to carry out these practical aspects of their relationships with patients requires a deeper level of interaction that involves not only CIPS, but an integration of their knowledge across several domains, for example, physical, social and psychological. From a broader counselling perspective, Egan's (2014) skilled helper model complements the discussion so far. Egan's model, which can be conceptually linked to Rogers' core conditions of genuineness, respect and empathy, is a framework that nurses can use to better conceptualise the helping process. It constitutes a map and set of techniques for exploring and managing relationships, which can be adjusted to meet individual adjustments to situations as they arise. There are three simple questions to address when using the model.

- What is going on?
- What do I want instead?
- How might I get to what I want?

Each of these questions relates to a stage in the model that can be followed sequentially but that may be used at any time. To answer any of the questions, the individual who is seeking answers tells his or her story and then explores with the helper ways to examine the options and solutions to the questions. The process involves looking at information and clarifying meanings. Early on in this chapter we talked about interpretations and perceptions and how they can exert influence. This model is a way of exploring in detail what individuals want from healthcare interventions and how nurses can assist them to gain these, as well as exploring some of the realistic options to achieving better health outcomes (see useful websites at the end of the chapter for links to the model for further study).

Activity 3.2   Decision making and critical thinking

Access the website:

www.gp-training.net/training/communication_skills/mentoring/egan.htm

Familiarise yourself with the website in relation to its aim, which is to use Egan's skilled helper model to help you in more effective problem management.

Choose either to work on your own, in relation to one of your own problems, or with a student friend in relation to his or her problem, or in relation to a problem experienced by a client or patient with whom you are working.

Work your way through the stages of the model, referring to the notes provided for each stage.

Later, consult Egan's (2014) *The Skilled Helper* book in relation to your activity notes.

Patients as decision makers

In the last decade, in the context of the emergence of contemporary respect paid to the idea that patients and service users are 'experts by experience', the government launched the *Expert Patients Programme* (EPP) (GOV.UK, 2013). This was in response to the evidence that more people in the twenty-first century are living into their 70s, 80s and beyond. The implications are that they will be living with long-term conditions and multiple pathologies. The programme is aimed at patients to enable them to self-manage their conditions and has a central tenet that, from the vantage point of their lived experiences, patients understand their disease better than healthcare staff.

The nurse's role emerges as enabling patients to find ways to solve difficulties and issues they have with their lifestyle and healthcare regimes so that they can feel and be more in control of those. Self-management programmes are run from local community centres. Nurses in acute and primary care settings can work in conjunction with this philosophy by adopting Egan's model, thus providing a framework to assist patients in decision making about their care. Lorig et al. (2008) evaluated the online EPP scheme and found that the programme appeared to decrease symptoms and improve health behaviours, self-efficacy and satisfaction with the healthcare system.

Chapter summary

In this chapter, distinguishing between the concepts 'risk' and 'safety', we have explored the meaning of being safe and effective in interpersonal relationships in healthcare. We also considered the relevance of social thinking models as explanatory frameworks and explored the many roles in practice, and the potential for role confusion. We identified a process for communication and interrelationship skills in healthcare settings. Finally we clarified what is meant by the helping relationship and the roles of both nurse and patient in this.

Further reading

Egan, G (2014) *The Skilled Helper: A problem-management and opportunity development approach to helping,* 10th edn. Belmont, CA: Brooks/Cole.

This book contains a lot of information on helping relationships, and will be a useful resource for Activity 3.2.

Grant, A, Leigh-Phippard, H and Short, N (2015) Re-storying narrative identity: a dialogical study of mental health recovery and survival. *Journal of Psychiatric and Mental Health Nursing,* 22: 278–286.

This is a relational autoethnographic study of the tensions that exist between mental health professionals and policy discourses and the lived experiences of survivors of the institutional psychiatric system.

Useful websites

www.gp-training.net/training/communication_skills/mentoring/egan.htm

This website gives information on helping relationships.

www.watsoncaringscience.org

The website of the Watson Caring Science Institute contains information on Watson's transpersonal theory.

Chapter 4

Understanding potential barriers to the safe and effective practice of communication and interpersonal skills

---

NMC Standards of Proficiency for Registered Nurses

This chapter will address the following platforms and proficiencies:

Platform 1: Being an accountable professional

At the point of registration, the registered nurse will be able to:

1.14 Provide and promote non-discriminatory, person-centred and sensitive care at all times, reflecting on people's values and beliefs, diverse backgrounds, cultural characteristics, language requirements, needs and preferences, taking account of any need for adjustments.

Platform 2: Promoting health and preventing ill health

At the point of registration, the registered nurse will be able to:

2.2 Demonstrate knowledge of epidemiology, demography, genomics and the wider determinants of health, illness and wellbeing and apply this to an understanding of global patterns of health and wellbeing outcomes.

Platform 3: Assessing needs and planning care

At the point of registration, the registered nurse will be able to:

3.9 Recognize and assess people at risk of harm and the situations that may put them at risk, ensuring prompt action is taken to safeguard those who are vulnerable.

Introduction

This chapter explores some main factors that may act as barriers and impede effective communication and interpersonal relationships. First, we investigate the shift we make in our professional work from social to professional relationships. The chapter considers how to develop safe professional relationships, by examining the different degrees of intimacy between friend and carer, and the rules of social engagement.

Next, we consider the effect that emotions can have on communication and interpersonal relationships. Emotions are clearly vital to communication; demonstrating our emotions to others enables them to recognise how we feel and tune into our emotional needs. This is made more complex by the need to balance our emotional expressiveness both with the need to construct new ways of coping with situations and with the extent to which we express or repress our emotions. Emotions can therefore both enhance and impede communication.

Other barriers to communication covered in this chapter include how we construct and interpret meaning in communication. The effect of motivation on communicating health advice is also explored. Finally, we consider the nature and some common forms of interpersonal conflict, how these arise, along with strategies to diffuse them in healthcare situations.

Shifting from social to professional relationships

The shift from social relationships to professional relationships requires a transition. This is from early social relationships based upon kinship or friendship networks to ones based on professional values and governed by a code of practice. These values encompass a sense of purpose, mutuality, authenticity, empathy, active listening, confidentiality and a respect for the dignity of the patient.

This requires nurses to do their best to manage their biases, prejudices and frequently their own emotions, even though these aspects of them as people are important as they bring to the encounter the humanness that is crucial to a sound professional relationship. The boundaries between social and professional relationships have arguably become increasingly blurred with the advent and increasing use of social media (see Chapter 5). For the moment, to help you differentiate between social and professional relationships, Table 4.1 compares some of the major elements of social and professional relationships. We will be exploring more of these elements as we go through the chapter.

Social	Professional
• You have no specific legal or professional responsibility for the person	• A professional has the responsibility for helping the patient regain a state of health; this involves a spectrum of activities that range from the physical to the invisible. This is governed by a professional *Code of Professional Conduct* (NMC, 2015)
• You may be related or have a code of behaviour that is either explicitly or implicitly agreed between a group, community or culture that provides a framework for sanctioning different codes of behaviour	• There is informality and formality in different settings and contexts
	• The patient and professional have to negotiate and agree the levels of formality on an ongoing basis, as dictated by work setting and goals
• Social engagement can be more informal in some instances and formal in others	
• The purpose of the relationship is not necessarily specific or geared towards particular goals	• The focus of the relationship is on the needs of the patient; often engaged through necessity rather than choice
• The individuals know each other through choice, social or family connections	• The behaviour of the professional will be planned, implemented and evaluated in a more formal manner
• There is often an element of spontaneity about engaging in the relationship	• The participants may not know each other
	• The participants may not like each other
• Feelings of liking, loving or fondness are involved and often expressed	• The professional seeks to be non-judgemental and non-partisan

(Continued)

Table 4.1 (Continued)

Social	Professional
• Persons are often judgemental within the social codes of their communities or family groups about those who are beyond those groupings and may share these judgements to gain a sense of consensus in the group of group or community characteristics	• Sharing of personal or intimate factors is mostly unidirectional from the patient to the professional • Confidentiality is a key factor in the professional relationship
• The feelings between persons in a social relationship may enhance or may detract from the relationship course	• The main aim of the professional is to work with patients to help them achieve a better understanding of the factors that are affecting their health and wellbeing, and co-facilitating their resolution • The feelings of the patient are identified, acknowledged and accounted for in any discussions • The feelings of the professional are woven into the encounter in the attempt to respond empathically • It may not be appropriate to express deeper personal feelings. This is a time for careful judgement by the professional. If extreme feelings are experienced by the professional it is important to seek professional support
• The sense of control in the relationship is more evenly shared or driven by the wants and desires of those communicating • The relationship may continue indefinitely or end depending on the degrees of mutual liking between the persons	• There is usually a planned ending to the relationship as a result of the resolution to the above factors • The professional has self- and professional knowledge through skills and education that are deliberately brought to bear on the encounter • The professional takes main responsibility for setting the boundaries of the relationship

Table 4.1 Comparison of social and professional relationships (adapted from Arnold and Boggs, 2006)

Becoming over-involved

One of the concerns professionals have is how to become involved with patients in a sufficiently supporting manner without losing objectivity through becoming over-involved. Being ourselves and bringing personal characteristics to the relationship is crucial, otherwise we would become mechanical, like robots giving care. The difference is that a professional relationship, which does indeed travel a fine line between compassion on the one hand and being so close that there is an over-involvement of emotional

investment on the other, has to draw a line between the two.
most likely to happen when a nurse feels an emotional conne
him of a situation or person from the past (this is called 'trar
or when there are shared feelings on a topic with the potentia

Another source of over-involvement is when a nurse feels g
tionship in which matters were left unresolved. This could
or a professional experience. The nurse may attempt to res
make the situation feel better than the earlier one, but the da

not regard the specific needs of the patient being cared for now. Often it will be an unconscious drive of which the nurse will be unaware. It may be others who notice the nurse is transferring her or his feelings from a previous situation to the one that is now being experienced. It takes a sufficiently self-aware person to recognise that these feelings are related to a different situation and to set them aside so that the patient's needs become uppermost. It also takes a professionally astute colleague to recognise what is happening.

Case study: Caring towards the end of life

Mary is a 79-year-old woman who has severely debilitating arthritis and is cared for in a nursing home. She is a quiet, placid woman who is widowed and has five children. Although they live some distance away, they all visit regularly, especially her two daughters and their children, who are now adults. Mary is a warm and kind person who is loved by her family. Her days are long and filled with pain from her arthritis and yet her mind is still alert and she loves to chat with the nurses. She can no longer move about on her own. She has a urinary catheter for her elimination needs, but requires regular enemas to help evacuate her bowels as the side-effects of the pain medication mean she is always constipated. She puts up with her discomforts valiantly, but the nurses are noticing that she is slowly becoming more sleepy each day and less interested in conversing with them. These are her twilight years.

It is very easy to become attached to this gentle, uncomplaining woman. She may be like the grandmother you wish you had, or even the grandmother you had and lost. If you did not have time to say goodbye to your own grandmother, your relationship with Mary could be even more poignant for you. It is in this kind of situation that you have to retain your professional distance and yet still strike a balance between caring and becoming over-involved.

We have already looked at endings in this book. In situations like this, endings need to be carefully and sensitively construed to avoid reliving previous emotional situations or experiencing regrets and guilt. In these kinds of circumstance, it is advisable for nurses to talk through their feelings with their mentors, clinical supervisors or colleagues to help them gain a sense of proportion.

...ting relationships with colleagues with whom you can share your feel-
...tuations or relationships is a strategy that will ensure that you are being
...toring or supervision by senior staff are also effective methods for support-
...f who are dealing with complex situations where there are no simple solutions
...gens and Heathershaw, 2013).

Activity 4.1   Critical thinking

Have a look at the following and mark on each line a point where you believe
the statements represent either social or professional behaviours.

	Social —— Professional
I am happy to joke with patients	←————————→
I am always smiling whatever is happening	←————————→
I would not let a patient cry; it does no good	←————————→
I think it is best to show your feelings all of the time	←————————→
I let people tell me as much as they want me to know	←————————→
I tell people exactly what I think of them	←————————→
I let people know that there will come a time when they will leave, so that we both know what to expect	←————————→

Hint: This activity will help you to distinguish better between professional
and social behaviour and also to reflect critically on aspects of your own
behaviour that you may take for granted.

Degrees of intimacy

There are two aspects of intimacy in CIPS practice. One is the physical space between
persons in an interaction, known as proxemics. The other concerns the degree to
which we disclose our inner feelings and thoughts to another, and the extent of self-
disclosure required in a relationship to achieve a greater depth of intimacy and
understanding between the partners. Both have relevance to understanding the relative boundaries expected in social and professional relationships.

Proxemics

Although there are cultural factors which qualify and complicate what follows, Hall
(1966) pioneered the study of proxemics and identified four spatial distances that

also correspond to types of social relationships. They are intimate, personal, social and public.

These four distances can be further divided into close and far phases. The far phase of one level can blend into the close phase of the next level. This will depend on the situation and degrees of comfort felt by individuals and also the shift from one distance to another, either to increase or contract the distance.

There are different ways to make theoretical sense of spatial distances. First, it is clear that individuals hold a buffer of space around them that acts as a protection zone against unwanted attack or touching. As nursing often takes place within this zone, it is important to consider how we move into this close proximity and reduce the sense of threat that this closeness may generate. Another theoretical position is that we strive to maintain equilibrium between varying degrees of intimacy and interpersonal relationships and adjust the spatial/relationship ratio accordingly. When the degree of equilibrium you have chosen is threatened, you may make adjustments, such as avoiding eye contact on a crowded bus or turning away.

The final theoretical explanation is derived from responses where individuals find themselves having their expectations of proximity 'violated'. Called the 'expectancy violation theory', it holds that, in these situations, the topic of conversation becomes less important and the overall status of relationship comes into focus in its place. Those who violate expected spatial relationships are judged to be less truthful. Yet, if you are perceived positively (i.e. of high status or particularly attractive), you will be perceived even more positively if you violate the norm. If, however, you are perceived negatively and you violate the norm, you will be perceived even more negatively. It is a minefield in which nurses have to tread very carefully so as not to violate the expected distance.

A good way to avoid such violation is to seek permission from the patient before carrying out a personal procedure and wait for a response before continuing. This may not be possible in an emergency situation, but it is always advisable to explain to the patient what you are doing and why. This will enable the patient to be more aware of your actions; even a semi-comatose person can hear a voice. Similarly, the tone and pitch of your voice, which should be gently questioning and not commanding, can provide reassurance. Informing and negotiating consent to invade a patient's personal space demonstrates respect for that individual's privacy and dignity.

Self-disclosure

How much do you tell patients about yourself to gain a sense of closeness in your professional relationship and to equalise the reciprocity between the information that you have about them versus the amount they have about you? Creating this balance is seen as a fundamental human need. First, let's consider what we may mean by 'self'. The work of Hargie (2006, 2016) points to the usefulness of considering nine different types of self, as shown in Table 4.2 (previously discussed in Chapter 2).

Me as	Type of self
I am	Actual self
I would really like to be	Ideal self
I used to be	Past self
I should be	Ought self
A new person	Reconstructed self
I hope to become	Expected self
I'm afraid of becoming	Feared self
I could have been	Missed self
Unwanted by one or more others	Rejected self

Table 4.2 Types of self

Activity 4.2 Reflection

Spend a few minutes going through the different facets of self in the first column of Table 4.2 (Me as) and see if you can describe yourself in each one. As you are in transition at the moment, as a student hoping to become a qualified nurse, you may find it easy. If you do not, you may wish to ask a close friend or family member to help you. Do you agree with the corresponding description of 'types of self'? Remember, these activities are not compulsory, so do not feel you have to complete the activity if it makes you feel uncomfortable.

Hint: This activity is solely intended to help you develop reflexivity about your own self (very important, especially in relation to role transition and socialisation into nursing).

Self-disclosure means communicating information about yourself. It may involve information about your values ('taking is not as important as giving love'), beliefs ('I believe that the world is square'), desires ('I would like to fly to the moon and back'), behaviour ('I eat sweets all day long') or self-qualities or characteristics ('I am always happy'). It is a natural part of interpersonal communication and can be verbal or non-verbal. In the former, it can be voluntary, or as a response to information from another person. In the latter, it can manifest itself in the clothes you wear or the way you speak. It can be best seen in the professional nurse–patient relationship as a developing process in which information is exchanged over a period of time, and which changes as the relationship develops from initial contact to more intimacy, perhaps to eventual deterioration, and closure.

Self-disclosure can be about facts or feelings. When meeting for the first time it is likely that the interaction will be about facts. In this circumstance, while you would not be expected to reveal facts about your intimate personal details, you can reveal facts about yourself to equalise the balance, for example how long you have been a nurse or worked on the unit.

It is accepted in relationships that there is a gradual progression from lower to higher levels of self-disclosure. However, in the professional nurse–patient relationship it has to be accepted that this is not necessarily the case. As deeper levels of disclosure are expected from the patient, the nurse's responsibility is to reassure the patient of the confidentiality related to the assessment and establish levels of trust, respect and confidence in the assessment process so that the patient feels comfortable with what will be an imbalance in reciprocity. A major factor is explaining why the information is needed.

Rules of social engagement

In most social situations, we know how to behave because we have learned the **social rules** that govern or guide the interactions. We have also learned from our regular involvement with activities and events – such as attending lectures, participating in handovers on the unit or having a meal out – the parts we have to play, such as student, staff or friend. This familiarity with social interactions, and the anticipated verbal responses and behaviours gives us a sense of security. We know what to expect, but in new situations where we might not know the 'rules of engagement' or have an understanding of the shared representations or intersubjective knowledge of what to do, we can feel anxious and isolated. We have to search for clues, observe behaviour patterns or listen to exchanges of information from those already established in the group. This applies to students on their practice learning experiences for the first time and for patients newly admitted or receiving care for the first time.

Research summary

In seminal work in a study investigating student nurses' occupational socialisation to nursing, Melia (1984) found that socialisation processes were linked to workplace rules. Social pressure from staff and other students on wards helped to enforce behaviours that, while acceptable to ward staff, did not always put the interests of the patients first. Melia found that, in order to fit in, students adapted to the new environments by not accepting either the education or general service view of acceptable practice. Instead:

(Continued)

(Continued)

Their main concern was to meet the expectations of those with whom they worked, especially those in authority.

(Melia, 1984)

The students thus viewed their training as a series of hurdles to overcome in order to survive. Does this apply to you today or have things changed?

Once local social rules have been learned, people can work and cooperate with a minimum of negotiation. This shared knowledge not only allows us to take familiar social situations for granted, but also makes any kind of adaptation or change to less familiar ones difficult, challenging and even threatening. Not only do we not know how to behave in those, because we are so accustomed to behaving in a certain manner, but we associate familiar situations with a central perception of ourselves that is also challenged. Our notion of who we are and what role we have to play is compromised, which may cause a profound sense of disequilibrium.

Patients clearly experience this disequilibrium when they enter healthcare settings. Understanding their perspective and enabling them to have a clear view of what is expected and the role they have to play can reduce anxiety and make communication more effective.

Making work-setting rules explicit can also help. For example, rules forbidding smoking are explicit. Rules for rewarding or punishing behaviours that are perceived to be unacceptable or do not conform to the shared social rules are not so explicit (Grant et al., 2015a). This is why patients and clients rarely ask questions – because they are wary of breaking an implicit work-setting rule and do not know what the sanctions will be if they do (Short, 2011).

Goffman (1959, 1972) was a seminal investigator of the social psychology of human interaction rules, who contributed greatly to our understanding of these in relation to managing the impressions others have of us, 'reading' interpersonal events correctly, and face-saving. Because of the complexity of these rules, we sometimes cannot avoid frequently breaking them. However, Goffman (1972) advised how we can minimise resultant damage, while convincing others that can be trusted, and are competent and worthy, through the judicious use of three social repair strategies:

1. Offer an account of why the error happened and give an explanation. This shows that no one is to blame and the error could not be helped – 'I needed to see the other person first because she was just about to go off duty.'

2. Offer an apology that accepts part of the blame. This is also an implicit promise that no harm was intended, that you are aware of the rules and that you can be

trusted not to transgress again – 'I'm sorry. I don't know why I did that. I knew immediately afterwards that it was wrong.'

3. Reconstrue the behaviour as one that was not breaking any social rules, but was part of another activity – 'I was only joking.'

However, there are times when these strategies are insufficient because the transgression is too serious, and it is likely that sanctions and damage will follow. In these circumstances, gaining support from colleagues is needed to approach the situation in a professional manner with a plan of action to remedy the situation as much as possible. Explanations and apologies are required to those who feel injured by the mistakes. Avoiding effective dealing with such mistakes will lead to unresolved guilt on the part of the perpetrator and potential repeated incidents of misunderstanding and mistrust.

The emotional context of communicating

Catherine Theodosius (2008) argues that the practice of nursing is a form of emotional labour. In taking this stance, she is encouraging nurses to engage positively with the fact that they cannot avoid the impact of their own emotions, or those of their patients, in nursing practice. Theodosius asserts that nurses should strive to make emotional labour therapeutic:

> *Therapeutic emotional labour (TEL) is therefore where the nursing intention is to enable the establishment or maintenance of the interpersonal therapeutic relationship between nurse and patient in order to promote the psychological and emotional wellbeing of the patient in a way that facilitates their movement towards independent health living. TEL is dealing with emotions that are directly concerned with expressions of self-worth and personal identity of both the patient and the nurse, elicited from their interactive relationship ... TEL may involve giving patients appropriate information on which they can act ... TEL may involve the nurse encouraging the patient to express and talk about their feelings and concerns while managing their own emotions. It is predicated on the belief that disclosure and discussion of personal and private problems is therapeutic for the patient and, within nursing, is typical of emotional labour represented in the Nightingale ethic. TEL may involve both the nurse and patient accepting the inevitability of death, predicated on the belief that the nurse can facilitate the patient towards as peaceful and dignified a death as possible.*

(Theodosius, 2008, pp146–147)

Just as for our patients, our emotions are a fundamental part of our personal identity. They are a mixture of pre-programmed (genetic, nature) and learned (social environmental, nurture), and can be demonstrated in many different ways through our actions and interactions. The phrase 'being emotional' is often used negatively about someone who is displaying an overtly emotional reaction to a situation by crying, shouting or being upset. Yet we do not always have to display our emotions to know that we are feeling them. Emotions can be either overt or hidden in the depths of our beings.

Sometimes we are aware of our emotions and sometimes we are not. This all adds up to fascinating, but complicated, phenomena in the human psyche. Emotions are also connected to the positive or negative values we place on objects, persons and situations. Thus, emotions can colour our perceptions of events and add a layer, or filter, to our experiences, which is intended to help us either cope with the exciting, demanding, unfamiliar and unpleasant, or understand the gravity or danger of an experience. Equally, our emotional state can sometimes lead us to impact negatively on our patients, in ways often outside our awareness. This is illustrated in the following case study.

Case study: Two very different nurses

Alistair spends a couple of days in hospital, in order to have a septoplasty procedure carried out on his broken nose. Two student nurses interact with him in relation to routine tasks that have been assigned to them. One is consistently cheerful and friendly with him, and helps him see the funny side of having what feels to him like 300 yards of gauze up his right nostril. From her facial expression, the other nurse always looks miserable and distant. She never speaks with Alistair and appears to him as if she would rather be on another continent. After the cheerful one disappears, presumably at the end of her shift, the occasional ministrations of the miserable-looking one begin to make Alistair wish that she was on another continent.

Emotions allow individuals to experience sensitivity and compassion for another, even though they might not fully understand the situation. As discussed, the emotions we feel in nursing practice are important; they are an inevitable part of how we respond and react to the persons in our care and to each other. As illustrated by the case study, caring for someone with feeling is qualitatively different from caring for someone in a distant and dispassionate manner. We utilise the information we receive about how a person is responding, whether it is with happiness, sadness or fear, to judge how we manage the interaction and carry out therapeutic interventions. If a person is very fearful of a procedure, the explanation and management of that procedure will require specific tuning to that person's needs. If another is experiencing significant loss or grief over a change in status or disfigurement from a wound, a nurse will adjust the care plan to take into account these feelings, in order to support and enable adjustment to the change in circumstances. A relative or friend who is angry and behaving aggressively because they believe treatment has not been timely or appropriate – often the result of miscommunication or a sense of lack of control – will need sensitive acknowledgement of their fears, worries and frustrations by the nurse, and the time to assimilate new information.

Balancing emotions

Our aim in life is to have a healthy balance of emotional experiences. This involves letting go of feelings that are damaging, and searching for new ways of dealing with situations that provoke unwanted emotional responses. This is complicated when individuals are unable to express their emotions, which may in turn be a function of not knowing what emotions they are feeling due to confusion, unusual circumstances or other changes to their status quo. Alternatively, people may know what they are feeling but not understand why, or may be experiencing conflicting emotions about the same situation. The nurse's role in these circumstances is to help patients clarify and identify their feelings with the aim of enabling a healthy expression or outlet for the feelings. One of the best ways to do this is to:

- understand the underlying reasons that have provoked the emotional response;
- allow the person to tell his or her story;
- identify and acknowledge the emotion that is being labelled in the story, for example, 'It must be frightening not to understand what is happening to your body right now';
- ask to help in a non-reactive way, which demonstrates caring by helping to obtain the needed information and validate the fears;
- identify if the person needs a break from the intensity of the situation, for example by arranging to come back later to talk over concerns again.

All these actions are key to developing an understanding and appreciation of the emotional context of a situation from the patient's perspective.

Case study: Coping with bereavement

Alicja, a first-year student nurse, begins a practice learning experience on a ward where there are elderly patients. She is suffering from unresolved grief over the recent death of her beloved grandmother. The ward staff notice she is finding it difficult to interact with the elderly women on the ward. Her mentor, a staff nurse, sensitively talks with her about this. When she finds out the reason behind the student's difficulty, she also hears that Alicja has carried her grief alone, without sharing her feelings with anyone. Alicja agrees to talk with her sisters and parents about how she is feeling, and within a couple of weeks she is able to interact positively with the elderly women on the ward.

Harmful emotional expression

Emotions can be harmful when they block adjusting to new situations, get out of control or affect another person by reducing self-esteem. Unresolved feelings can lead to communication misunderstandings in which needs are not perceived to be met. Feelings perceived to be unacceptable can be hidden behind a mask of calm or rationality. Repressed feelings can be expressed with an excessive intensity that is disproportionate to the situation. Consequently, communication and relationships can be distorted by misperceptions created through emotions that are unexpressed, overexpressed or inappropriately expressed. Therefore, the feelings about the content of an interaction have to be balanced with the feelings about what is happening to the self or others in any situation (Hargie, 2006, 2016).

Some barriers to communication and interpersonal relationships

Before considering common barriers, it is relevant to review the aims of communication and initiating relationships in the healthcare context. We hope your reading of this book so far has prepared you better for more effective interactions, specifically around:

- establishing a trusting and respectful relationship;
- transmitting and sharing information;
- exchanging ideas and understanding perceptions;
- creating a platform for renewed understanding;
- enhancing understanding of attitudes, ideas and beliefs;
- achieving mutually acceptable goals.

An essential ingredient for interactions to be effective is for meanings to be shared and understood. To do this, meanings must be checked and awareness heightened around blocks to communication that can arise as a result of the many differences between individuals. These include differences in relation to authority, power, language, ability and disability, personality, background, gender, health, age, race and socioeconomic group.

Meaning

Communication can always be enhanced through identifying and working through barriers. Exploring meaning, which is an active process created between participants in an interaction between source and receiver, speaker and listener, writer and reader, can help identify some of those barriers. Meaning is not only dependent on messages but also on the interaction between the messages, the thoughts and feelings within those messages, and on the assumptions underpinning them. Consequently, meaning is not just 'received'; it is co-constructed or built up from messages heard or read and combined with social and cultural perspectives, for example beliefs, attitudes and values. The more the understanding of the meaning is shared, the less likely it is to lead to a breakdown in communication.

Activity 4.3   Reflection

Below are five topical concepts and a potential rating descriptor. Consider each concept and place your own descriptor/word that represents the meaning you have for that concept in the graded column that represents your strength of feeling along a continuum of good to bad. Compare your sense of meanings with a peer.

Concept	Good 1	2	3	4	Bad 5
Abortion					
Terrorism					
Social inequality					
Brexit					
Climate change					

No two individuals are likely to derive exactly the same meaning of the above concepts and, because people change their views and ideas about life, it is not always possible to predict accurately another's sense of meaning. Indeed, your own meanings may change from one day to the next depending on your experiences. To refine this process as much as possible, verify the perception you have of another's meanings by asking probing questions, echoing what you perceive to be the other's feelings or thoughts, and seeking elaboration or clarification. As a general rule, it is wise not to assume that the meaning you attribute to phenomena, actions, situations, behaviours and emotional responses will correspond with someone else's.

Conflict

There are times in every relationship when those involved will agree to differ. Misunderstandings arise when conflict is experienced and it's assumed there is something wrong with the situation or the relationship is in jeopardy or damaged. Differences of opinion where two sets of thoughts or ideas differ are not unresolvable. The situation that develops into an aggressive outburst is one where the issue has expanded to include personal egos, lack of trust, and emotional perceptions resulting in an increasing misrecognition of the situation. The role of the nurse in such situations is to be aware of the dynamics and the skills required for their resolution, and put those into practice.

Frequent conflict can serve as an alarm to indicate that a relationship needs closer attention. The disadvantages of conflict are increasing negativity, hurting others and depleting energy that is needed for other emotional tasks. The positive effects are that it can lead to a closer examination of issues that are developing in a relationship or group. Examining the problems and finding solutions to the conflict can be a way of mending bridges and strengthening relationships. Nonetheless, experiencing conflict can be disquieting and uncomfortable, giving rise to feelings that can be challenging or in opposition to closely held beliefs or values.

The first step in conflict resolution is to analyse the situation. In line with the work of Arnold and Boggs (2015) it is useful to consider:

- previous experiences with conflict situations;
- the degree to which the conflict is acceptable;
- the intensity of the feeling it arouses;
- the physical, cognitive and emotional health or stamina of the persons involved;
- the subjective interpretation of the event or conflict;
- the consequences.

Conflict can become manageable when the causes, sources and issues underpinning the conflict are clearly articulated by the parties involved. This needs time and the use of non-judgemental listening skills to collect the stories. By drawing out hidden feelings or repressed ideas that otherwise may not have been known, barriers to communication can hopefully be identified and resolved.

One of the most common responses to conflict is anger. It originates in a part of the brain called the amygdala, which is responsible for thought and judgements. The anger

---

Theory summary: Aggressive behaviour

The human response to conflict is defensive, and defensive behaviour can also be aggressive. Aggressive behaviour can take three forms: aggressive, passive and passive–aggressive responses.

- The aggressive response is to deflect potential or actual attack through attacking or blaming someone at a personal level. This triggers anger, resentment and counter-aggression in the person being attacked or blamed.
- The passive response is self-preservation through not engaging in or attempting to resolve interpersonal conflict. This generates feelings of frustration in the passive responder and loss of respect for her or him.
- The passive–aggressive response is where, on the surface, a person appears to be agreeing to plans and arrangements that are made, but in reality is not engaging with the activities designed to solve the problems. There can be verbal agreement at the same time as sabotaging or discrediting activities undertaken by the passive–aggressor, which leads to confusion and mistrust.

response is intended to identify threats and prepare our bodies for attack. This rapid response is very necessary in life-threatening situations; however, it does not always give us time to think about appropriate responses or the consequences of our actions.

Activity 4.4   Team working

With a group of peers, identify the sources of conflict that you have witnessed in the clinical areas you have experienced so far. Separate out those situations that involved staff to staff, staff to patients, patients to staff, and patient to patient. Analyse these situations to identify common features of the causes of conflict.

What examples have you witnessed of good conflict management? Compare these with poorly managed examples.

Hint: This activity is aimed at helping you start to develop your skills in conflict recognition and conflict management. Often conflicts are allowed to fester and grow in healthcare environments, usually to the detriment of patient and client care.

The second step in conflict resolution is to identify the potential solutions to the problems or issues that are causing the conflict. Key elements for any professional involved in a conflict situation are to remember that the rights of the individuals involved are to be respected and to behave in an assertive manner. Assertiveness needs to be learned and the websites listed at the end of the chapter will provide you with some resources to work through. Before setting up a conflict-resolution meeting, again drawing on the work of Arnold and Boggs (2015), consider the following:

- *Prepare for the encounter.* Be clear about the purpose, the major points to discuss and whether the information you have is complete and can be shared. Give careful consideration to the language used and the choice of words so that messages are clear and unambiguous.
- *Organise your information* and consult with another to validate your approach, preferably someone who is objective. Rehearse.
- *Manage your own anxiety.* Use breathing and mindfulness techniques to calm you help you maintain emotional equilibrium.
- *Time the encounter.* Judge when parties will be receptive, allow time for discussion and expressions of choice and be prepared to listen.
- *Take one issue at a time* and focus on the present. Break the problem down into small units or steps and allow time for clarification. If one small area can be resolved, this can lead to further resolutions.

- *Request a change* in behaviour or response. Assess the level of readiness and take into consideration maturity, culture, values and life factors.
- *Evaluate the conflict resolution.* It may take more time; small goals can be achieved first. Aim for a climate of openness and future communication.

Taking steps to solve problems and reduce conflict requires skilled handling and can be achieved through observation and practice in role play.

Chapter summary

In this chapter we have explored some key relationship boundaries between professional relationships and friendships/kinships. We have looked at the implications of rules around intimacy and proximity. Emotions, and how they need to be balanced to achieve effective communication outcomes, have been discussed and you should now understand the construction of meaning and how this underpins communication messages. We have stressed the importance of interpreting meanings to clarify understanding and perceptions of events. You have learned how motivation factors can affect health messages, and how to identify common benefits and barriers to achieving health-promoting communications. We have also explained common forms of conflict and provided some suggestions for how they should be handled in healthcare settings.

Further reading

Arnold, E and Boggs, KU (2015) *Interpersonal Relationships: Professional communication skills for nurses,* 7th edn. London: Elsevier.

A key text that further clarifies some of the issues raised in this chapter.

Theodosius, C (2008) *Emotional Labour in Health Care: The unmanaged heart of nursing.* London: Routledge.

An excellent primer on the role of emotion in the work of nursing, including the practice of CIPS.

Walker, M and Mann, RA (2016) Exploration of mindfulness in relation to compassion, empathy and reflection within nursing education. *Nurse Education Today,* 40: 188–190.

This article looks at the viability of the inclusion of mindfulness into the nursing curriculum.

Useful websites

www.businessballs.com/self-confidence-assertiveness.htm

This website has information on assertiveness training.

www.mentalhelp.net/poc/center_index.php?id=116&cn=116

This site about anger management has many resources explaining the physiology and psychology of anger as well as techniques for managing angry outbursts.

www.breathworks-mindfulness.org.uk

An excellent resource site for mindfulness information and training generally and in healthcare contexts.

Chapter 5 The learning and educational context of communication and interpersonal skills

NMC Standards of Proficiency for Registered Nurses

This chapter will address the following platforms and proficiencies:

Platform 1: Being an accountable professional

At the point of registration, the registered nurse will be able to:

1.17 Take responsibility for continuous self-reflection, seeking and responding to support and feedback to develop their professional knowledge and skills.

Platform 2: Promoting health and preventing ill health

At the point of registration, the registered nurse will be able to:

2.2 Identify and use all appropriate opportunities, making reasonable adjustments when required, to discuss the impact of smoking, substance and alcohol use, sexual behaviours, diet and exercise on mental, physical and behavioural health and wellbeing, in the context of people's individual circumstances.

Platform 5: Leading and managing nursing care and working in teams

At the point of registration, the registered nurse will be able to:

5.8 Support and supervise students in the delivery of nursing care, promoting reflection and providing constructive feedback, and evaluating and documenting their performance.

Chapter aims

After reading this chapter, you will be able to:

- describe how to integrate theory and practice;
- understand the importance of learning from experience, so that learning can be based on reality;
- understand the role of communication in health and health promotion, including digital and social media communication;
- appreciate that you have a role as an educator;
- manage reflection in portfolios for assessment;
- identify activities to enhance communication in learning and teaching situations;
- commit yourself to lifelong learning.

Introduction

You will have many learning goals in your time as a student and this chapter will guide you in achieving these through enhanced CIPS practice. So far in this book we have been focusing on CIPS for your role as a professional. In this chapter we will focus on how CIPS can support you and your individual learning pathway – now and throughout your career. The way we will do this is to look at a spectrum of your role as learner through to educator, and your own continuing learning needs as a lifelong learner (Figure 5.1).

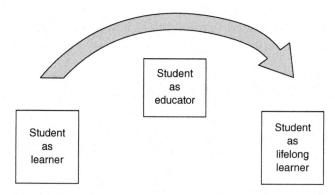

Figure 5.1   Spectrum of learner, educator and lifelong learner

This chapter will examine each of the three stages in the spectrum, beginning with a discussion on you as a student and learner. We will explore some of the issues related to the integration of theory and practice, leading to a discussion on how learning should be realistic and relevant to your practice and learning needs. One way to achieve this is through experiential learning techniques, which we will explore by deconstructing the concept of learning. Learning through experience is regarded as learning by doing, rather than by listening to others or reading. This form of learning involves active learning through interactions, increasing self-awareness, expression, flexibility and reciprocity. Learning *through* experience (which refers to deliberately planned learning experiences) and learning *from* experience (which refers to past experiences to gain new insights) are two highly relevant learning approaches in CIPS.

After a brief look at the role of theory to practice evidence portfolios, we will explore learning styles and what makes for skilled performance. We will then turn to the role of the student as educator. This will include the importance of your engagement with digital and social media communication, and your credibility as educator and health promotor. The chapter will end with an exploration of the meaning, significance and implications of lifelong learning for you.

The student as learner
Integration of theory and practice

One of the constant dilemmas for nursing students during their studies is the need to integrate theories learned in the classroom with the practice of nursing performed in clinical, real-world situations. This is no easier with CIPS, which can seem so obvious and yet, as this book demonstrates, are not just simple skill sets to be learned in a rote fashion. We all have CIPS abilities and what has to be achieved during studies is enhancing, improving and making more effective these skills in healthcare settings. We have already explored some theories in this book and have attempted to use practical exercises to demonstrate how the theory can be applied. Judging how meaningful these are and how they can be applied to good effect helps with the integration of theory with practice. But it may not be enough.

The NMC *Future Nurse: Standards of Proficiency for Registered Nurses* (2018) asserts that practice, integrated with theory, needs to be evidence-based, and thus safe. In Chapter 2, we explored the importance of integrating theory with practice and the relationship to research that provides the evidence for safe practice. As with any practice-based skill, practice makes perfect and this applies equally to CIPS. Practising using the skills by working with models in a safe environment is as essential as rehearsing clinical skills. The difference may be the self-consciousness or self-awareness you may experience as you say words that are unfamiliar or use phrases that, at first, sound false and stilted. The conditions you need in order to practise are therefore important.

Disconcertingly, there is continuing evidence in the last two decades that final-year nursing students and newly qualified nurses have difficulty sustaining the values and ideals they gained during their training (Jasper, 1996; Maben et al., 2006, 2007a).

Activity 5.1 Reflection

What are the ideal conditions that you need in order to practice a new communication or interpersonal skill?

Do you need to be alone and in front of a mirror? Or do you need to be with a close friend, or in a group? Each of these situations can pose different levels of complexity in communication, how you use your interpersonal skills and the feedback you will get on the effectiveness of your skills.

Hint: This activity will help you increase your awareness of your CIPS learning style. It will help you learn about practice situations that inhibit you, compared with those in which you feel more relaxed. Generally, it is a good idea to proceed from relaxed to increasingly inhibiting situations.

There is a consensus around the fact that while nurses may gain a strong set of values and ideals during their programmes of study, there are professional and organisational factors that work against them realising these values and ideals in practice. One major reason for this can be found in the damaging contradictions between the explicit nursing undergraduate degree curriculum and the implicit 'way things are done around here' curriculum that nurses are socialised into in their practice organisations, both before and after they qualify (Grant and Radcliffe, 2015).

There are of course unavoidable additional demands, such as time pressures, constraints on roles and role development, staff shortages and work overload. In addition to the ideal-retarding effects of service organisations, these demands constitute the fact of twenty-first-century healthcare working environments. However, practising and applying CIPS ideas, concepts and theories during and beyond your course will enable you to play your part in closing the never ending theory–practice gap.

Learning for reality

Eve Bendall (1976) was one of the first nurse researchers to study the theory–practice gap. In her seminal work on how students learn clinical skills, she found that students described one thing in writing and then did something completely different in practice. At the time, the 1970s classroom assumption was that a written description by a student nurse would be sufficient evidence to judge that the nurse was competent to carry out care for specific patient conditions. Her study found this assumption to be false and was pivotal in formulating the practice-based curriculum that nurses experience today. However, nursing practices must always be contextualised in psycho-social contexts, so it is unsurprising that since the 1970s what constitutes these practices has qualitatively changed. They have expanded from purely physical activities with, for example, visual, auditory, verbal, tactile, kinaesthetic and organisational factors, to include those underpinned by the social and human sciences (Bendall, 2006; Goodman, 2015b). This is apparent throughout this book, and most explicitly in Chapters 8 to 11.

There are different views about how best to enable nurses to learn practical skills. One view is that principles should be taught early in the course, so that they can then be taken into practice settings and applied and practised in different situations until competency is reached. In this approach, the practice of such principles is supervised by a qualified mentor and then assessed.

Another view is for students to observe care being delivered and for its elements to be identified by students. So, for example, in a ward or community setting, the nurse carries out different actions with and for the patients. The task of the student is to make note of these activities and assemble them into a whole picture of care that is required for that particular setting. Once assembled, students follow up the tasks to discover whether there is evidence underpinning the activities, and prioritise and discriminate between their essential and unessential elements in preparation for carrying them out without supervision. This is a more complex and detailed method, requiring placement mentors to establish whether or not students have been successful.

Each of these approaches has advantages. With regard to the first, this is that students are prepared with ideas and strategies before they enter the practice setting. Many students find this comforting, as they do not wish to be seen as incompetent when they find themselves working with patients. It also enables students to feel more confident about potentially confidence-undermining situations. The second approach is based on the idea deriving from **gestalt** psychology that all experiences are based on the sum of the individual parts and that, by examining the parts, a whole can be assembled with better understanding of how the parts interact.

Experiential learning

A third approach to practice learning is through experiential learning. This model, proposed by Kolb and Fry (1975), assumes that exposure to a nursing experience is accompanied by observations, reflections, cognitive and emotional processing, and practice, in a four-stage learning cycle, represented in Figure 5.2.

Kolb and Fry's model has been further adapted to include the processes of reviewing data and information that will happen during thinking about the experience. The next stage is to puzzle out or give some meaning to the experience. This is then added to the ideas that will influence any further experiences or responses to situations (Figure 5.3). The main premise is that we all have an intrinsic tendency to draw upon our experiences of the world we live in, to improve our knowledge of what happens to us, formulate our opinions and extend our range of skills and knowledge.

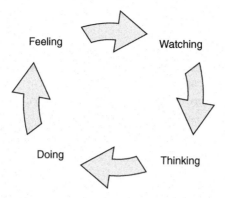

Figure 5.2   A simplified version of Kolb and Fry's experiential learning model

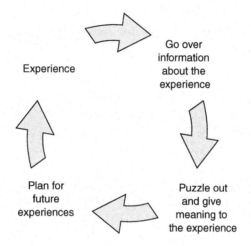

Figure 5.3   Experiential learning cycle

Using experience to guide our actions and beliefs does, however, present its challenges. If our current reactions are based solely on previous experiences, this may inhibit our future learning through reducing our response flexibility. We are never in a position where our accrued experiences will prepare us sufficiently for the next challenge; thus wisdom based only on past experience is limited. We need to be open to learn from new situations.

Decisions to base our actions on previous experiences are always founded on assumptions, whether 'true' or 'false', and either our conscious or unconscious assimilation of ideas. It is the stage of the cycle where we ascribe meaning to events and experiences. By interpreting the experiences, and attempting to understand why something is happening, we use different strategies to give an event meaning. Meaning can be drawn from the symbolism of an event, when a particular event might have more significance to some than to others, such as attending the memorial service of a loved one. Meaning can also be drawn from a moral or psychological sense of purpose.

For example, 'If I work hard and qualify as a nurse, I'll be able to make an important contribution to the world.'

We rely on our previous experiences to guide our responses but do not necessarily learn from, or adjust, our responses to improve on how we react in situations. Most of the time we place our memories of experiences in 'cold storage' or classify them as 'unfinished business', to be returned to when we have enough psychological energy. This explanation can help us understand why some people never seem to learn from experience, because they never sufficiently return to the cold storage of their memories. This points to the essence of experiential learning. It is not just learning to do something differently next time, but is more about actively engaging in an analysis and reflection on what has been learned, how it compares with previous learning and how this accumulative store of learning can be built upon further to improve skills and knowledge for future situations. This is so relevant when learning about CIPS. You will have already stored up many experiences of your own and will have also refined some of your interpersonal skills as a result of those experiences.

Activity 5.2   Reflection

Take a moment to think about a communication misunderstanding that you have experienced. Now consider what you learned from that experience. What was your interpretation of it? How would you improve your communication of information in that experience the next time you face a similar situation?

Hint: This activity, if practised regularly, will help you engage in the experiential learning cycle described in Figure 5.3, better preparing you for future communication encounters.

In nursing, students are given time to learn in practice under the guidance of mentors or experienced healthcare practitioners. In the same way that you learn to carry out a physical procedure, it is important first to observe communication and interpersonal interactions. You can then practise under supervision and be prepared to undertake communication of information on your own. At each stage of the process, you will continue to learn and you will need to create opportunities to review what you are learning, clarify what you have learned from past experiences and think about future experiences to extend your skills. So that you can also gain optimally from these experiences, it is important to know when you are learning by experience as distinct from learning from experience.

Learning by experience is more or less an unconscious process. It is a realisation after the experience that we have learned something significant. These experiences are gained through the realities of professional life, varying and unpredictable demands and changing circumstances. An example of this is that we are often fearfully preoccupied with getting something right, and when we forget to try, and get it right anyway, there is a sudden integration of knowledge and surprise that the skill can be mastered after all.

To get the most out of these experiences, you need to hone your skills of attention to both external events and what you are experiencing internally. Internal processes include noticing your thoughts, intuitions, emotions, bodily sensations, intentions for yourself and others, needs, what you are doing, how you are doing it and how all this relates together (Figure 5.4).

Learning from experience is more deliberate and conscious. The intention is not just to experience the 'here and now', but to devise future actions based on the reflection and evaluation of events.

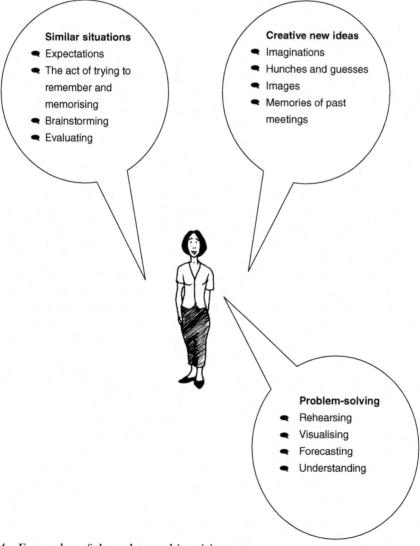

Figure 5.4 Examples of thoughts and intuitions

Using the experiential learning cycle (look back at Figure 5.3) requires time for thinking and reflection. Some of this goes on informally in social groups or at the end of a shift with groups of peers. The more aware we become of our feelings and intuitions about experiences and the comparison of these reflections on both inner and outer experiences, the more helpful our memories of the experiences will be. By practising using the experiential cycle, students can integrate it to the extent that they begin to work through its stages automatically. This serves to enhance their reflections and learning through experience to greater effect.

Assessment of practice in portfolios

Bearing in mind that you need to demonstrate a wide range of thinking skills alongside your development of practice skills, there remains the thorny issue of how both theory (which is an intellectual activity related to your thinking skills) and practice can be captured in one place to demonstrate the achievement of competence. One method is by using portfolios of evidence. Since the early 1990s, portfolios have been used to capture evidence of nursing students' learning in practice. Over the years, these have been consistently developed and improved from initially being bulky repositories for sheaves of paper to slimmer versions providing a succinct method for collating evidence. They have now become an integral part of the majority of nursing education programmes (see Reed and Standing (2011) for further guidance).

Learning styles

There are several theories on learning styles, with most focusing on three or four main attributes. Two of the most widely used are the learning-style inventories of Kolb (2000) (whose experiential learning theory we examined earlier in this chapter) and that of Honey and Mumford (1992). Both of these versions can easily be found on the internet for you to test out yourself (see useful websites at the end of the chapter). Essentially, Kolb's inventory suggests that we each have a preference for one of four styles: concrete experience (feeling); reflective observation (watching); abstract conceptualisation (thinking); and active experimentation (doing). These are clustered into two continua with conflicting axes: feeling and thinking versus watching and doing. Kolb believes that we choose to learn by grasping at an experience to transform it into something that is meaningful and useful. Our learning styles are therefore a product of either preferring to watch and do, or think and feel.

Honey and Mumford believe there are also four dimensions to learning styles. They describe these as characteristics and divide people into activists, who learn by doing; reflectors, who stand back and observe first; theorists, who prefer to adapt and integrate experiences into a conceptual whole or framework; and pragmatists, who, while on the lookout for new ideas, will only adopt ideas if they have a practical benefit. There are some similarities between Kolb's and Honey and Mumford's approaches to learning styles, but you may want to ponder over which approach best captures your own.

Identifying your preferred learning style will help you recognise the work you will need to do on other areas of the dimensions described above, in order to become more reflective. If, for example, you recognise that you are primarily a pragmatist or 'doing' learner, you may wish to work at developing your capacity for observing, thinking and feeling. Such practice should result in an improvement in your approach to reflection as a learning strategy and in you having a more positive outlook towards this form of learning.

Skilled performance

While you may now realise that experiential learning, reflective writing and your preferred learning style may influence how you achieve your learning goals in the assessment of your practice, you will want to know what makes a skilled performance stand out when practice is being assessed. Some essential characteristics are outlined in Table 5.1.

Accuracy	**Skill executed with precision**
Speed	Movements are swift and confident
Efficiency	Movements are economical, with the ability to draw upon additional movement when required
Timing	Timing is accurate and the sequential order is correct
Consistency	Results are consistent, and repeated successfully on different occasions
Anticipation	Can anticipate events very quickly and respond accordingly
Adaptability	Can adapt the skill to current circumstances
Perception	Can obtain maximum information from a minimum of cues

Table 5.1 Essential characteristics of skilled performance

Any skill has to be practised before it is learned. The more you practise your communication skills with colleagues and friends, and think about the different situations that require different responses, the more this will help you refine your skills and improve your confidence. You are also advised to hone your observational skills and make notes of situations in, for example, the classroom, waiting rooms, clinics and in practice. Evaluate these interactions and conjure up scenarios where you might improve your skills. By developing the skills of observation and analysis, inviting feedback and considering the context in which nursing practice takes place, your critical reflection skills will also develop and you will avoid any negatively framed, overly introspective analysis.

The student as educator

You may regard yourself as a student who is there to learn rather than teach. However, there will be frequent opportunities when you will find yourself giving an explanation, directions, instructions, a presentation, or untangling a misunderstanding, and you will be – in effect – teaching others some aspect of healthcare (Arnold and Boggs, 2015). This could be teaching a fellow student either in the practice setting or in the classroom, explaining their health issues to patients or clients, or presenting a project you have undertaken as part of your studies to qualified staff. We live in exciting times, when the co-production and dissemination of new knowledge between student nurses and their lecturers is encouraged (see e.g. Grant and Barlow, 2016; Grant et al., 2016).

Seven top health communication skills

Because there are so many factors affecting communication between healthcare professionals, and between those professionals and patients or clients, it is difficult to refine the competencies into a 'laundry list'. However, seven top health communication skills have been distilled from a range of different research studies and are outlined briefly here.

1. Giving accurate and sufficient feedback

Feedback is a message sent back to the message sender to give reassurance that the message has been received and understood. For example, it is reassuring for patients or clients to receive feedback that they have been understood, or for you to receive reassurance from them that they have understood you. Also, don't be afraid to give positive feedback to colleagues to encourage further good performance. Too often, healthcare staff believe themselves to be continually caught up in punishment dialogues, with their positive contributions to their jobs ignored.

If you are uncertain whether something has been clearly understood by your nursing, medical or other healthcare colleagues, ask for confirmation, or ask if any further explanation is required. Alternatively, if you see an inaccuracy in performance, or poor performance, do not be afraid to bring this to the attention of qualified staff.

Non-verbal feedback is equally important, as it registers reactions to what has been said in, for example, facial expressions such as surprise, boredom or hostility. Non-verbal behaviour needs to be in synchrony with verbal messages, to minimise the risk of 'double' or conflicting messages. As described in the previous chapter, our non-verbal behaviour can sometimes give away our emotions and preoccupations when we are least aware of this, no matter what we say verbally, often to the detriment of our relationships with our patients or colleagues. Even apparently innocuous behaviours, such as leaving the room or remaining silent, are non-verbal communications that may give negative signals to, or alienate, those we care for or work with.

2. Listening attentively

This means actively attending to what is being said and how it is being said. It is listening without making judgements or letting your own perceptions act as a barrier to what is being said by the other person. It requires giving signals that you are actively listening by using appropriate prompts, such as 'mmm', 'I see', 'how interesting' or 'OK', and non-verbal prompts, such as nodding and smiling, and also giving feedback to show that you understand what is being said or conveyed. Such *active listening* indicates that you are working hard to understand the other person, and enables trusting relationships, rapport, mutual interest and understanding.

Activity 5.3   Communication

Arrange two chairs back to back. Have a friend sit on one chair and yourself on the other. Have the friend tell you about a journey they have just taken. Let them speak for a couple of minutes. Do not interrupt your friend or ask any questions. When your friend has stopped, recount to them what they told you. Then place the chairs facing each other. Sit opposite your friend and ask them to tell you about their day at work for two minutes. Again, do not interrupt or ask questions. When they have finished, relate back to them what they have recounted to you.

Compare the two experiences from two points.

* How did it feel to listen and not speak?
* Did you remember more from the first or the second task about the events?

Hint: What pass for 'normal' social exchanges are often 'duologues' rather than dialogues, with one person waiting for the other to stop talking so that s/he can start talking. In that kind of encounter, neither person listens to the other properly. Practice in this activity should help you experience what it's like to listen carefully and attentively, and will stand you in good stead to develop the practice of active listening with your patients and colleagues.

3. Interpreting accurately

In interpreting what at first appears to be dubious information voiced by a patient or colleague, it is important to avoid immediately forming a prejudicial opinion on what has been said. Instead, a careful assessment of the extent of the other person's level of understanding may be required. To this end, it is also useful to collect any cues from non-verbal information and assess the extent of this influence on what has been said. To make this estimation, you will use as your baseline your own experience or level of knowledge and expertise about the situation or condition. It is then possible to make a judgement or evaluation on the accuracy of this understanding, which can then be utilised, for example to help a patient gain further understanding of health advice on weight management or to improve accuracy of a procedure in the case of a fellow student. Therefore, interpreting means gathering information before you form a judgement and explanation of a situation or events, with the intention of improving understanding.

Interpreting messages is also a form of translating, and you may be called upon to translate from one language to another. A frequently occurring example of this is changing the bioscientific terms used in medicine into everyday language, to enable understanding or meaningful comprehension on the part of patients. It could also involve taking a complex idea and transforming it into a simpler and more understandable idea that is related to the real-world situation of the patient or setting.

4. Giving clear instructions

This is a skill that requires practice and is harder than it seems. One way to become accomplished is to talk through what you are doing as you are carrying out an activity, and (this is most important) say why you are doing what you are doing.

As a general rule, when working directly with patients, always begin with the simplest explanation and work towards the more complex. This is invaluable when you are carrying out procedures with patients whom you require to participate but who may be anxious. In these situations gradual exposure to information is needed so that their anxiety is not further increased by information overload, and information should be paced according to patients' information needs. However, when teaching a skill to colleagues, a different tack is needed whereby all the information will need to be transmitted; yet this can also be in a graded and staged approach to facilitate assimilation and retention of information.

5. Behaving in a professional manner

Nurses have a legal and moral duty to maintain their competency and to work within the scope of their practice. There is an expectation that nurses will act in a professional manner, and establish realistic boundaries related to time, purpose of the interaction, and level of involvement with patients and those in their care. These principles also relate to interactions with fellow students and nursing and other healthcare colleagues. Intrinsic to these principles are notions of respect for basic human dignity, cultural openness, sensitivity to individuals' circumstances, an understanding of the impact of ill health or disability, and an adherence to standards of care. Conveying these attributes to colleagues and patients is an important part of demonstrating your professional awareness and competence. A further consideration is the use of research evidence to improve nursing practice, which can be integrated into your educator role through, for example, patient information on health-promoting activities and informational presentations for colleagues.

6. Communicating information clearly

The first step to communicating clear information is to know your audience and what they will accept as a preferred means for messages to be communicated. Questions to consider are: which language is being used (jargon or lay terms), what dialect is needed (nurses need to switch from one form of language to another in relation to dialect or generation), whether humour is acceptable, the extent and limits of confidentiality, whether the messages should be personalised, whether learning styles are an important factor to consider, and whether a different style is required for children, adults with learning difficulties or aggressive patients.

The next step is to decide whether the message is task- or relationship-oriented. An example is the instructions given by flight attendants before take-off. If humour is injected to gain your attention, are you annoyed, as you believe it trivialises the information, or does it make you sit up and listen? The task is the inclusion of information about safety procedures, whereas the relational aspect is the inclusion of personalised remarks that could either reduce or exacerbate tension. You will have to decide which approach to use by knowing your audience. There will be times when the task is the most important aspect of the communication, perhaps in emergency situations, and there will be other occasions when the more relational aspects will be paramount.

When all these factors are considered, the appropriate message medium can be selected to transmit the information. Selection of message medium now, of course, includes the use of contemporary information technologies as well as written and verbal models of message transmission.

As part of the NHS reforms in 2011, the government set out to consult on how information is communicated via different technologies to patients in *Liberating the NHS: An information revolution* (DH, 2011). It has been part of the government's agenda to create a 'put patients first' giving people more information and control, and greater choice about their care. Since August 2014, the NHS has been concerned to provide information that meets an appropriate Accessible Information Standard (NHS England, 2014a). More attention is being paid to how information is given to patients and in formats that are understandable and accessible. A more technical approach is from the development called Patient OnLine (NHS England, 2014b), which is intended to promote online services to patients, including access to records, online appointment booking and online repeat prescriptions.

Increasingly nurses need to consider their role in how technology is used to communicate messages, and this may involve learning new skills with contemporary and developing technologies. Nurses need to learn 'digital professionalism' (Ellaway et al., 2015; Jones, 2016; Jones et al., 2016) as social media platforms such as Twitter and Facebook bring both new possibilities and new risks involving confidentiality and the public display of your 'private' attitudes and behaviours (in the mental health nursing context, see Leigh-Phippard and Grant, 2017).

This is an opportunity for nurses to take the lead in developing **informatics** skills. On an individual communication level you will need to think about assisting patients in navigating and understanding information resources to enable more self-care via sources such as the internet (Jones et al., 2015). For your own development you will need to embrace 'digital professionalism' (Jones, 2016; Jones et al., 2016) to use information technology resources proactively to keep up to date with current practice, such as telemedicine, telenursing and remote nursing (for a selection of resources on new developments in this field, see useful websites at the end of the chapter). You will be expected to access and use patient clinical diagnostic information to inform clinical decisions and to use information to help deliver more effective care, in order to meet quality standards and audits of clinical care.

7. Establishing credibility

As a student, you may believe that you have little credibility as an educator, yet credibility can also equal believability, which is the ability to inspire belief or trust. You may wish to consider how you could demonstrate these characteristics to others in a manner that may not rest solely on your nursing knowledge, but more on the kind of person you are or are becoming. In the early stages of your course, you may feel unable to take on the responsibility of teaching others. However, as you progress through the programme, even moving from one year to the next, you will be in a position to help more junior students with advice and information.

Credibility is also about your acceptability among your colleagues, and demonstrating that you can be reliable or helpful can generate acceptability. The perception that a person is competent, knowledgeable and skilled enhances credibility. Demonstrating these characteristics in areas where you have proven your ability, such as through examinations or presentations to your colleagues, is particularly effective in strengthening interpersonal relationships.

Case study: Sarah's presentation

Sarah is coming to the end of her second year. Although she is anxious, she wants to consolidate her practice learning experience with a presentation of what she's learned to her nursing and other healthcare colleagues. She uses Microsoft Office PowerPoint to help make the presentation seem as professional as possible, while balancing this with lively and appropriate images she's downloaded from the internet.

The presentation goes very well. She receives positive feedback about it from all of her colleagues which gives her confidence to do this more often in the future.

Communication and health promotion

Earlier in this chapter we proposed that a student has the opportunity to become an educator in many different situations. One that is becoming increasingly important is as an advisor on promoting health and wellbeing. The World Health Organization (2000b) called for the explicit inclusion and application of health promotion in all nursing curricula. Twelve years later a study by Walthew and Scott (2012) demonstrated that student nurses had difficulty in understanding the concepts of health promotion and health education and that they used information-giving techniques without any notion of empowering individuals to understand their own health needs. The text *Health Promotion and Public Health for Nursing Students* (Evans et al., 2014) explains in detail the concepts involved in understanding empowerment and would be useful further reading.

Evans and colleagues suggest that, when talking to people about health matters, you need to think how you will translate jargon or technical language into language that can be understood, without seeming patronising. The key in this situation is to find out what the person already knows and what s/he understands, to build on this. From here you can clarify and explain any unknown terms and provide correct information where there are misunderstandings. This step-by-step approach helps to forge a partnership between you and the person you are trying to help. It is also important to divide the information you provide into manageable 'chunks'. Too much information can overload anyone, especially if they are feeling unwell or anxious, and these states of mind can also affect a person's retention of information. If you introduce a stepwise approach to the conversation patients will be able to absorb the information and nurses can facilitate deeper learning (understanding) as opposed to patients simply memorising superficial information (surface learning).

The student as lifelong learner

The NMC *Future Nurse: Standards of Proficiency for Registered Nurses* (2018) stresses that nurses should commit themselves to lifelong learning, and think in a future-directed and nursing field-related way. This idea was first articulated by Basil Yeaxlee and Eduard Lindeman in the 1900s, when education was proposed as a continuing aspect of everyday life (see Falk, 2014). The notion of learning throughout life is not new, as a peep into Plato's *The Republic*, written nearly two and a half millennia ago, reveals. Initially, lifelong learning was deemed to be for learning's sake, and therefore non-vocational. However, in recent decades, a gradual shift has taken place in which lifelong education has been reconceptualised as lifelong learning. The world we inhabit has seen rapid economic, social and cultural change in recent times, towards 'knowledge' or 'informational' societies characterised by the never-ending need to keep up with technological and related societal developments. Consequently, many adults now take part in non-formal learning activities – short courses, study tours, membership of fitness centres and sports clubs, heritage centre activities, self-help therapies, life and lifestyle coaching, electronic social networks and self-instructional media.

The importance of skills

The increasing importance of skills in the UK population is seen as a major challenge when set against world economic forecasts for global economies. This may seem a lofty ambition, far removed from your studies as a student nurse. Yet, there are implications for you and your future working life; you will need to be aware of the continual demographic changes that are impacting qualified practitioners in the health field as well as people in all walks of life.

In the wake of Brexit, the UK is facing an uncertain economic future. As our population continues to age, there is demand for high-level skills, with rapid changes in technological developments, locally and globally. We are relying more and more on innovation to drive our economic growth, and our national productivity trails many of our main international competitors. The UK has high levels of child poverty, poor employment rates for the disadvantaged, regional differences in income and other forms of inequality (Wilkinson and Pickett, 2010), especially inequalities in health (Marmot, 2010; Dorling, 2015) A current and future workforce of increasingly skilled nurses is crucial in contributing a national response to these challenges.

Your future career path will be guided by many factors, ranging from your personal circumstances to your career goals and aspirations. You may wish to undertake further training to become an advanced or specialist practitioner, roles which are vital and well established in many fields of nursing. *Advanced-level nursing: a position statement* (DH, 2010) provides a benchmark that is generic in that it applies to all clinical nurses working at an advanced level, regardless of area of practice, setting or client group. It describes a level of practice, not a specialty or role, which should be evident as being beyond that of first-level registration. The benchmark is viewed as a minimum threshold. It comprises 28 elements clustered under the following four themes (as agreed by expert practitioners):

- clinical/direct care practice
- leadership and collaborative practice
- improving quality and developing practice
- developing self and others.

It should be clear to you now that, due to changes in technology and the corresponding moving frontiers of information, you will constantly be required to acquire new skills and knowledge. Lifelong learning will therefore be integral to your continuing professional knowledge and competence, including the need to continually develop your CIPS throughout your professional life.

Chapter summary

In this chapter, we have explored stages of learning opportunities for students. Rather than concentrate on the classical approach to study skills (which can be found in a number of excellent textbooks), we have chosen to discuss how students can integrate theory with practice. There is no doubt that learning for practice realities should be the goal for students of nursing. We have suggested this can be achieved by experiential learning and have provided a structure to develop this skill. Guidance on how to achieve a skilled performance has been provided for professional development. The role of the student as educator was explored, and advice has been given for achieving effective communication in healthcare settings. Finally, the relevance of lifelong learning, both personal and professional, has been examined.

Further reading

Arnold, E and Boggs, KU (2015) *Interpersonal Relationships: Professional communication skills for nurses*, 7th edn. London: Elsevier.

Evans, D, Coutsaftiki, D and Fathers, P (2014) *Health Promotion and Public Health for Nursing Students*, 2nd edn. London: Sage Publications.
Two useful texts for teaching health promotion and health education.

Leigh-Phippard, H and Grant, A (2017) Freedom and consent. In: Chambers M. (ed.) *Psychiatric and Mental Health Nursing: The craft of care*, 3rd edn (pp. 191–200). London and New York: Routledge.

A useful chapter for considering issues around empowerment through social media communication, for nurse, service user and other stakeholders in healthcare communication.

Useful websites

www.businessballs.com/kolblearningstyles.htm

This site has details on Kolb's learning styles inventory, and a brief comparison with Honey and Mumford's variation on the theory.

http://resources.eln.io/honey-mumford-learner-types-1986-questionnaire-online/

This site will help you see what Honey and Mumford's learning type you fit into using a quiz.

Chapter 6 The environmental context of communication and interpersonal skills

Chapter aims

After reading this chapter, you should be able to:

- understand how different care settings might undermine the practice of safe and effective CIPS;
- describe the importance of material and social-environmental factors in the practice of good communication in healthcare and be able to identify examples of each, in relation to communication within and between groups, families and populations;
- understand what is meant by the terms **prejudice** and 'schema development' and their relation to language use in nursing;
- appreciate the demands placed on CIPS in British nursing by the nature of multi-culturalism;
- identify some of the ways in which institutional racism impacts on communication and interpersonal exchanges in British nursing practice and the ways in which healthcare organisations defend themselves from accepting that they may be institutionally racist;
- describe the meaning of the 'fallacy of individualism' as it pertains to CIPS practice in British nursing care.

Introduction

The environmental context of CIPS for nurses ideally includes multidisciplinary team practice, and intra- and inter-professional working, across different care settings, within, hopefully, safe environments. This chapter begins by introducing you to a discussion of the importance of CIPS within multidisciplinary team practice and inter-professional working, across different care settings and populations. A specific case study will be presented of sexual abuse within a care home. This is intended to help you recognise the relationship between a lack of safety and a breakdown in communication within a specific care environment.

The discussion turns to how environmental factors are key to shaping communication. With regard to the social environment, communication within and between populations, groups and families, and between young and older people, will be discussed and illustrated with appropriate examples. It will be argued that such communication takes place at conscious and unconscious levels simultaneously and utilises power to the advantage of some groups and the disadvantage of others.

Next, we help you explore the interrelated concepts of prejudice and schema development. These concepts (introduced in Chapter 2) have emerged from developmental psychology and, together with the role of language use, are extremely important in understanding how CIPS can break down in specific healthcare environmental contexts.

Then we discuss the impact of shifting friendship, family and cultural networks on communication and interpersonal behaviour and skill development. The demands on CIPS arising from the British multicultural society will then be contrasted with institutional racism, and its impact on communication, in healthcare environments.

The chapter ends with a critique of the tendency emerging from humanistic psychology to view CIPS as solely located within the individual. In the light of the preceding argument, this 'fallacy of **individualism**' will be argued as naive and conveying an overly optimistic picture of human agency and interaction.

Multidisciplinary team practice and interprofessional working

The demands of two or more professional groups communicating effectively within the same team are considerable. When environmental factors are added to the melting pot, the recipe for danger can increase in an alarming way. The following case study demonstrates a specific example of a phenomenon prevalent in recent years, and makes for disturbing reading.

Case study: Communication and sexual abuse of the elderly

On 25 February 2001, *The Guardian* newspaper reported an example of the sexual abuse of an elderly woman in a nursing home. In 1991, she suddenly stopped taking her medication. At that time, her family made the assumption that this behaviour was related to an inevitable progression of her slide towards Alzheimer's that had begun some years earlier. However, soon afterwards, she started to exhibit terror each time her formerly beloved son-in-law entered her room at her nursing home. Again, her family made sense of this in terms of her illness progressing very quickly.

It was only when the owner of the nursing home was arrested for sexual attacks on the elderly women in his care that the family began to piece together a number of strange incidents that had escaped their notice at the time. By that point the old lady had died. Her daughter was of the opinion that her mother wasn't listed as a victim in the court case because the authorities didn't seem to want to discuss what had happened. She further asserted that none of the people whose mothers were abused in the home knew what was going on.

The owner of the nursing home, a man in his mid-60s, was sentenced to four years in jail. That was in 1997. But it seems a cultural and statistical certainty that the sexual abuse of old people by care workers is still going on today.

Some years later, the director of the website and helpline Action on Elder Abuse (**www. elderabuse.org.uk**) expressed the view that sexual abuse of elderly people in care and nursing homes was extremely prevalent. She stated that the helpline received lots of calls from frantic families and care home staff concerning extreme sexual abuse in these homes, and was of the opinion that the number of calls grossly under-represented the true level of abuse taking place. She gave the view that individuals suffering from mental and physical frailty were perfect victims for such abuse, given that they can't defend themselves or get away from the environment they find themselves in.

She added that, in her view, such abuse was more about power than sex, and that there were even pages on paedophile websites encouraging men finding it hard to access children to gain employment at care homes.

Catalogue of assault

According to Action on Elder Abuse (2017), 'elder abuse' constitutes '[a] single or repeated act or lack of appropriate action, occurring within any relationship where there is an expectation of trust, which causes harm or distress to an older person'. There are five main types of abuse in care homes:

- *physical* – including hitting and restraining, or giving too much, or the wrong, medication;
- *psychological* – shouting, swearing, frightening or humiliating a person;

Activity 6.1   Team working and research

As a group doing an internet inquiry, investigate the extent to which any of the above is still prevalent or has changed for the better since the early 1990s.

- What safeguards are in place to protect the vulnerable?

Hint: The aim of this activity is to help you develop your skills in critical internet searching.

- *financial* – illegal or unauthorised use of a person's property, money, pension book or other valuables;
- *sexual* – forcing a person to take part in any sexual activity without his or her consent;
- *neglect* – depriving a person of food, heat, clothing, comfort or essential medication.

Teamworking

This topic appears a good deal in the leadership literature. The focus is on ensuring good team work to improve patient outcomes. There are *descriptions* about what makes a team (Katzenbach and Smith, 1993), what holds teams back from working effectively, how a team develops (Tuckman, 1965), and what the proper role for team members may be (Belbin, 1981). We also need to think critically about our teams in actual practice and whether there are parallel teams trying to exercise clinical or managerial leadership (Edmonstone, 2009, 2014). Culture, organisational development and notions of what leadership and management may be will affect how a team performs, and whether it actually is a team or merely a group.

Team dynamics can be influenced by many factors and working with other professionals can involve issues around hierarchy, gender and your 'reflexive deliberations' – the inner voices that direct your action (see Chapter 9).

Effective team building might be hampered by more than the individual characteristics each person brings to the team. For example, interprofessional barriers to both stages of development and the roles team players enact might be:

- sex role stereotyping;
- separate professional education;
- separate lines of management;
- business culture vs. care culture vs. cure culture;
- poor communication;
- differential status;
- lack of informal interactions;
- differing value systems;
- conflict.

Patrick Lencioni (2002) outlines five dysfunctions of a team – these represent the 'dark side' of our behaviours:

1. Focusing on personal success, status and ego before team success.
2. Ducking the responsibility to call peers on counterproductive behaviour which sets low standards.
3. Feigning buy-in for group decisions creates ambiguity throughout the organisation.
4. Seeking artificial harmony over constructive passionate debate.
5. Unwilling to be vulnerable within the group.

Lencioni (2017) argues that a key point is 'holding ourselves *mutually* accountable' (includes 'passing the buck' – or it's 'not my job/role'), a lack of which indicates a dysfunctional team. This means we need full openness, no avoiding and holding peers to account, which might make *the* difference in really high performing teams.

The King's Fund (Ham, 2014) have provided six case studies which illustrate effective team and inter team working. They argue effective teamwork is the fifth cultural characteristic which is fundamental to high quality care. Getting beyond *hierarchy* (alongside inspection and markets) is a key message.

One method to overcome ineffective communication between and *within* professional teams, and to try to overcome issues of gender and hierarchy, is the use of a structured process such as SBAR: 'situation, background, assessment and recommendation' (Thomas et al., 2009). SBAR has been found to be an effective way to improve communication among staff thus improving patient safety (Brewer and Jenerette, 2011; Drach-Zahavy and Nadid, 2015). A structured handover may actually positively affect mortality rates (Hudson et al., 2015). A standardised method should help focus attention on what is required, recognised and acted upon within teams, which should foster a culture of patient safety (NHS, 2008).

The environmental impact on communication

The importance of environmental factors in skilled interpersonal communication was argued in Chapter 3. To recapitulate, the environment is a very important factor in shaping communication. With regard to the elderly, for example, residential healthcare environments produce opportunities and constraints for staff and patients around communication. As can be seen from the above worst-case scenario of sexual abuse, communication between staff and patients, and between patients and their relatives, can be seriously compromised under conditions of extreme exploitation of patients.

The exploitative exercise of power in such a circumstance can stay undetected and unreported when staff, and some relatives, engage in selective attention, rationalisation and denial. This might be played out when people choose not to notice certain disturbing facts because it clashes with their interests. For example, nursing staff in a rest home may not want to recognise signs pointing to the home owner's serial abuse of residents because of a fear that 'going public' about this might result in them losing their jobs, and along the way becoming very unpopular with some of their colleagues. Conversations about the possibility of such abuse then become forbidden territory, although the uncomfortable, non-verbal behaviour of some nurses will be telling.

The material environment

The material environment is both physical and social. At the level of physical environment, the layout and shape of buildings can both provide opportunities for, and constrain, good interpersonal communication. In illustration of this, Nussbaum et al. (2000, p14) argue:

> *the architectural design of a nursing home can 'control' the interaction within the building. If the nursing home is designed with a central nursing station and has residential wings extending from the center, it is very unlikely that individuals who are placed in separate wings will enter into a relationship. Proximity is a primary factor for selecting an individual for interaction, and the architecture often dictates who will be close both physically and relationally.*

The social environment

Communication with and within groups, families and populations will vary in style, content and function. Researchers working in the related areas of social identity theory and self-categorisation theory argue that group norms influence behaviour when the social identities with which they are associated are meaningful to the individuals in the group (Hogg and Vaughan, 2011). Put more simply, people in different social and/or professional groups will experience social identities that 'work' precisely because other members in their particular group experience themselves as having similar or complementary identities.

Social identities will correspond to specific sets of attitudes, behaviour and communication styles, and, for some people, to **culture** and **ethnicity** (see Chapter 7). Their ability to adapt to their new circumstances is also likely to depend on the flexibility of their personal schemas (see Chapter 2), the strength of their social identity (which might be antagonistic to the new set of people they find themselves in), their mastery of the language used in the new social environment (see discussion on both of these topics below), their age, their perception of how safe they feel, and numerous other factors. We now consider these issues in the context of using CIPS with children, adolescents and teenagers.

Communicating with children

Nina Dunne

Getting the Right Start: The National Service Framework for Children, Young People and Maternity Services – Standards for Hospitals (DH, 2003, p16) states:

> *For children and young people to participate fully as partners in their care they have to have access to accurate information that is valid, relevant, up-to-date, timely, understandable,*

developmentally ethically and culturally appropriate. A range of communication methods should be developed and used ... in a variety of formats, media and languages.

Children have a right to effective communication in the healthcare setting. Indeed, the United Nations Convention on the Rights of the Child (United Nations, 1989, p4) asserts: *Children have a right to be consulted, to be heard, to express their own views and feelings.* Communication supports everything children's nurses do. Effective communication skills are therefore crucial in developing professional and therapeutic relationships with children and young people and this is embedded in the theory of family-centred care.

There is also a moral obligation to communicate effectively with children (Department for Children, Schools and Families, 2004; United Nations, 1989). They therefore need to be treated as active partners in the care that affects them, and be allowed to exercise choice and have the right to make decisions (Department of Health (DH), 2003). When children are treated as active partners in healthcare, adherence to treatment regimes can improve (Tates and Meeuwesen, 2001). Children also appear less upset and recovery rates improve.

However communication with children is generally a neglected area (Levetown, 2008), with some healthcare professionals continuing to describe children as beings who are not yet able to understand and communicate in an appropriate manner, and therefore unable to contribute to the therapeutic relationship (Tates and Meeuwesen, 2001; Favretto and Zaltron, 2013). Directly challenging such assumptions, very young children seem to be generally more accurate in providing information about their health status than their parents (Riley, 2004). Moreover, excluding children can cause them to experience a sense of abandonment (Clarke et al., 2005). Children's enhanced understanding provides a sense of control of the situation, and their perceptions of their value are important due to the relationship between their levels of self-esteem and self-worth and medical outcomes (Prilleltensky et al., 2001).

Communication difficulties

When communicating with children, you need to consider their developmental as well as their chronological age. The environment and situation will also affect the child's level of communication as anxiety and unfamiliarity can cause difficulties with communication. Many children can pick up on body language and facial expressions, and misunderstandings can occur if the child perceives a difference between what is said verbally and non-verbally. You therefore need to be aware of your own gestures and facial expressions as this can hinder communication.

When interacting with a child who has communication difficulties it is helpful to gain the assistance of the parent/s in interpreting what has been said. The use of interpreters and translators can confer both benefits and problems. Professional translators are aware of cultural issues and can diffuse situations where questions considered inappropriate for that culture have been asked.

Levetown (2008) has developed three elements for *physician–parent–child communication*:

1. *Informativeness*: quantity and quality of health information provided by physician.
2. *Interpersonal sensitivity*: affective behaviours reflecting the physician's attention to, and interest in, the parents' and child's feelings and concerns.
3. *Partnership building*: the extent to which the physician invites the parents (and child) to state their concerns, perspectives and suggestions.

In extrapolating from this to nursing practice, it is important information provision matches the cognitive needs and levels of the child and family and therefore you must be able to assess the developmental level of the child in order to communicate effectively. This forms the basis of healthcare professional *task-related behaviour* (Levetown, 2008, p1442).

Interpersonal sensitivity and partnership building address the affective needs of the patient and/or parent, thus focusing on their emotional needs. It is important the child and family feel heard and not just talked at. Feeling heard constitutes *relational behaviour* (Levetown, 2008, p1442) and partnership building is central to family-centred care and shared decision making.

Communicating with children of different ages

Teaching children how to communicate with healthcare professionals was found to be effective in seminal work (Lewis et al., 1991), which suggested children taught in this way preferred an active role in their care and felt they had a better experience whilst in hospital as a consequence.

Infants: birth to 12 months

In order to develop language skills, infants need exposure to speech and it is therefore essential that nurses talk to infants and toddlers and interact with them in order to stimulate them. Infants also need to be able to see the face of the person speaking to them and, as distance sight is still developing, it is important the nurse is close to the infant to maintain eye contact.

The tone of voice is also very important, and infants respond to a voice with both a higher pitch and a sing-song quality. Infants tend to communicate through coos, gurgles and grunts, although facial expressions and more extensive body language are also used. It is important the nurse is able to get the help of the parent when trying to interpret these sounds and movements. When you carry out interventions with children in this age band, it is important you talk through and describe procedures as you are doing them.

Toddlers: 12 to 36 months

Toddlers communicate with a combination of gestures, grunts, one- and two-word word sentences, positive and negative emotional expressions, and body movements. They can assign meanings to words. They do want to be able to express themselves, so patience on the part of the nurse is required. Parental involvement to help in interpretation may also be useful. The implication emerging from this for you is that, in the context of separation anxiety, you may be seen as a stranger so trust needs to be established first. Discussion and explanation of a procedure should occur immediately before its implementation.

Pre-schoolers: 3 to 6 years

Pre-schoolers begin to talk in full sentences that are grammatically correct. Young pre-schoolers may struggle with accounts describing events in the correct order, but by age 6, sequencing events comes much more easily. However, they can still easily misinterpret conversations and have a short attention span. In this regard, it is important you explain the procedure that is about to be carried out with reference to all the senses: that is, what the child will see, smell, taste, hear and feel, and that you are honest about the pain the child may feel.

School-age: 6 to 12 years

School-age children talk in full sentences, much like adults. They ask more questions, can relate past experiences in vivid detail and seek more information and justification for the way things are. Moreover, school-age children can handle receiving more pieces of information at the same time compared with pre-school children. All of this points to nurses using books and pictures to explain procedures. Children within this age band are developmentally ready to handle detailed explanations. However, it is important you do not patronise the child and ask children how much information they would like.

Some communication techniques

In attentive listening, the nurse pays attention to verbal and non-verbal cues in attempting to understand the content and the feelings behind the discussion. However, making assumptions about what the parent or child wants to say, judging the parent or child, and allowing the conversation to move off-track can be barriers to attentive listening.

Using silences can encourage parents to speak by giving them time to think through information and consider alternatives. However, silences should not be allowed to go on too long as this can become uncomfortable.

The use of questioning can help with clarification. Open questions allow the parents to respond in the way they choose and can encourage disclosure, but the conversation can move off-track. So questions should be focused and not too general. Closed questions can make parents feel they are being rushed and, although useful for clarifying information, they can also be leading.

Communicating with parents

Children's nurses need to communicate with parents as well as the child. Poor communication with parents can affect their recall and therefore adherence to treatment regimes (Hallström and Runneson, 2001). Parents need information that is timely even if it is distressing (Perrin et al., 2000). Some parents also want advice which can put the nurse in a difficult situation. Above all, parents want to feel they are being listened to. They also want to be involved in how their children are informed (Tates and Meeuwesen, 2001) and the amount of information their child is given. However, it is important nurses are mindful this may conflict with the needs of the child and can hinder the child's treatment and recovery. Enhanced understanding can provide the child with a sense of control.

Activity 6.2   Communication

As a group, work on the following scenario.

Three-year-old Alice has difficulty breathing and is showing signs of respiratory distress. She has laboured breathing and is obviously uncomfortable. Alice's observations are within normal limits; however her respiratory rate is 24 respiratory rate per minute. Her hands and feet are cool and pale. Alice's mother is quite tearful and emotional seeing her child like this. Alice's father is angry nothing is being done quickly enough to help Alice and is questioning everything you are doing.

- What is the goal of communication with the patient and parents?
- What are the challenges of communicating with the patient and parents in this situation?
- Would communication without the parents present help the situation?
- How will you achieve this?

Hint: This exercise will help you think through some of the complexities of working with children in this kind of healthcare scenario.

Communicating with adolescents and teenagers

Chris Cocking

As a qualified nurse you will routinely come into contact with adolescents and teenagers – young people – in clinical practice, whether or not you choose to work specifically in paediatric nursing. It is therefore vital you are able to communicate effectively with them.

Activity 6.3   Team working and reflection

In a group, before reading further, explore your attitudes towards teenagers and adolescents (you might be one yourself!). Identify the ways in which perspectives expressed are related to the ages of people in the group.

Twelve- to 18-year-olds are often categorised as a unified social group ('adolescents' or 'teenagers') that is feared and/or pathologised in society and popular culture. However, because it is a stage everyone goes through on their path to adulthood, it is important you build on your understanding of the physical and psychological challenges experienced and how this may influence individual communication styles and development. First of all, it's worth highlighting that not all scholars see this period of transition as an objectively fixed concept and Thurlow (2005) suggests the concept of adolescence is more of a social and economic construct than determined solely by age or biological changes. Furthermore, young people's categorisation as a single homogeneous group (e.g. 'teenagers') is often imposed upon them by adults. For instance, Williams and Garrett (2005) argue that young people may come to identify as a group at least in part because they are often uniformly treated as such a group by adults and their associations with their peers are often demonised and/or curtailed.

While young people's associations with each other and the resulting peer pressures they can experience are often considered as negative influences and responsible for a variety of negative outcomes (including involvement in gangs, and the development of eating disorders), their social networks can also be a source of support and strength that help them deal with the challenges of adolescence (Drury, 2015). There is evidence (Fortman, 2003) that young people rate communication with adults less positively than with their peers, and that this dissatisfaction is at least in part due to the perception that adults fail to engage effectively with them, which could explain why young people may be reluctant to communicate with adults.

Fortman suggested viewing adolescent communication and behaviour from an inter-group perspective would be more beneficial than merely looking at individual communication styles. Furthermore, in a review of adolescent communication with adults in authority, Drury (2003) argued that antagonistic representations of how adults view communication skills in young people (and vice versa) could contribute to a vicious cycle of poor mutual interactions, with adults considering that young people have poor motivational and communication skills, and young people highlighting the power imbalance and lack of respect that adults have for them as contributing to the communication difficulties they experience. However, merely framing the issue in terms of helping young people to improve their communication skills could also deflect responsibility from adults looking at possible deficits in their own communication. Therefore Drury (2003) concluded that any efforts to 'improve' young people's communication skills need to be considered in a broader context of unequal group relations.

Challenges in communicating with young people

The issue of communication has clear relevance for how young people engage with health professionals, and so it is vital for nurses and other health workers to consider how they engage with such a client group. Poor communication could not only reduce the effectiveness of health interventions if young people do not follow advice from professionals, but could also result in their avoiding engagement with health services altogether if they feel their needs are not being considered or understood. Wrate (1992) found that doctors perceived adolescent patients as sullen or even hostile, and it seems likely this could in turn affect how they then interacted with them, however good they believed their own interpersonal skills were.

A common cliché is that young people can be uncommunicative (any parents of teenagers may well be used to grunts, one-word answers, shrugging of shoulders and the term 'whatever' when their offspring talk to them!). However, the reasons for such communication difficulties are more complex than teenagers simply losing the ability to speak in words of more than one syllable. For instance, Drury et al. (1998) found that when young people reported communication difficulties with parents, this was because of a lack of a shared point of view or unwillingness to hurt parents' feelings. When looking at communication difficulties with their employers, lacking the courage to speak out was listed as a more common reason.

Therefore, if faced with an uncommunicative young person in hospital, rather than putting it down to typical teenage behaviour, it is worth trying to find out any possible underlying reasons for this unwillingness to communicate and seeing if you can help improve the situation. For instance, a young person admitted to accident and emergency may be scared, disoriented, in pain, or even unwilling to be there (especially if s/he has been brought in by an anxious parent). So, recognising the distress the young person may be in, and helping to devise strategies to deal with such fear and uncertainty could help improve effective communication. Giving the young person space to communicate without the parents present can also be useful if any parent–child dynamics are escalating the situation (although be aware that this can often require equally good communication skills with the parent when requesting privacy to communicate with the young person!).

Young people's use of language can be a source of mystery to adults and they often use phrases and/or slang that may appear strange, or sometimes inappropriate and grossly offensive. This places a demand on nurses to separate out what may be socialised usage of language by young people without them fully understanding its possible implications from conscious attempts to oppress others through the expression of prejudiced attitudes, and respond appropriately in both instances. The reasons for young people creating their own communication styles (and sometimes their own language) can be varied, but Fortman (2003) argued they often define themselves through how they verbally interact with others. This can be a strategy to maintain a positive sense of group identity that is different from adults, which is in line with Tajfel's (1982) social identity and Turner et al.'s (1987) self-categorisation theories from social psychology. These suggest that people seek positive self-esteem by categorising themselves into social groups with similar others with whom they identify.

A word of caution is necessary before you run off to learn the latest guide to teenage slang. Although it's good for nurses to understand and be able to engage with young people, it's also important to realise that they may resist adults using 'teenager language'. This is because part of the reason for its use is to gain positive in-group distinctiveness by communicating in a way that sets them apart from adults, as predicted by Tajfel (1982), and this process can be undermined by adults trying to re-appropriate their terms.

Cultural awareness

Since the majority of communication is non-verbal, there is more to communicating with young people than being familiar with the language they may use. Therefore, it is vital to be aware of ways that young people may communicate with others by culturally expressing themselves. There are currently a variety of youth subcultures in the UK (such as Goths, Emos, Metallers, Ravers, Skaters), each with its own style of clothes and behavioural norms that may influence how they interact and communicate with adults. Nursing staff need to be accepting of these different forms of cultural expression, and engage with the young person in a non-judgemental or discriminatory way, however bizarre or even offensive they may find the young person's dress sense or bodily piercings.

These subcultures can sometimes be linked to reasons why young people come into contact with health services, but this should not be allowed to influence your interactions negatively. For instance, Young et al. (2006) found that identifying with Goth subculture was strongly associated with deliberate self-harm and suicide attempts amongst young people in central Scotland, so nurses may need to be sensitive and non-judgemental when dealing with such clients who may present with evidence of deliberate self-harm.

If you find that you share some social or cultural interests with your young clients, this may be a way of initially engaging with them and can help encourage trust and the creation of a therapeutic relationship. However, you also need to be clear about the need to maintain effective professional boundaries, so you can present an appropriate role model to sometimes impressionable and/or vulnerable clients, and don't find yourself in awkward situations with them or your colleagues. For instance, younger qualified staff and/or student nurses who find it easier to identify with the young people they work with could be perceived as being a softer touch than older/more senior staff, and so more susceptible to attempts at manipulation.

Case study: A hypothetical scenario

Vicky is a 22-year-old newly qualified nurse who identifies as being from the Goth subculture. She has just been offered a job working with young people aged from 12 to 18 in an inpatient unit. She passed the interview with flying colours, but was told by the local manager that she needs to present herself as an appropriate role model when working with vulnerable clients, and this means that when working on shift, she should dress appropriately and remove any facial piercings for her own safety. She also used to self-harm by cutting when she was 15 or 16 to help cope with a depressive episode she experienced after being bullied at school and has long scars down her arms (although she hasn't self-harmed since). It has been agreed that she can disclose her own experiences of self-harm if she thinks it will be helpful for her to develop a sense of empathy with particular clients who are otherwise difficult to engage with, and/or as a therapeutic tool to show that it is possible to come through such episodes and develop other forms of coping. She has been advised that she needs to exercise good judgement in this matter, and be aware of the need to maintain appropriate professional boundaries. Therefore, it has been agreed that she will cover the scars on her arms when working on the ward and/or in groups, but is allowed to reveal them during one-to-one sessions with clients if she considers it appropriate.

Think about the benefits of following this approach and any possible challenges that Vicky might experience from clients and/or other colleagues.

Communicating via technology

It is worth discussing the technology young people use to communicate with each other and how it may affect nursing practice. Given the explosion in young people's use of IT devices and social media, parents could be forgiven for thinking that their teenage children are unable to survive without being in constant contact with their peers via the latest device that is in vogue. Nursing practice needs to keep up with such advances in communication technology, and most clinical environments now have policies on the use of mobile phones while in hospital (NHS, 2009). In some Child and Adolescent Mental Health Service inpatient environments, young people may be allowed to keep their mobiles with them while admitted, as they could be a useful way to keep in contact with the outside world, to reduce feelings of isolation and/or homesickness while in hospital. However, staff may also reserve the right to regulate their use if they have any concerns regarding possible safeguarding issues arising from their use. For instance, young people often swap numbers with each other on admission in an effort to make friends within the new social group, and unfortunately peer dynamics sometimes mean that people fall out with each other and bullying by text could happen when adolescent friendships break down.

Disclosure

As a nurse, you will often be interacting with young people when they are removed from their natural environment, which can result in confusion and fear for them. However, this can also be an opportunity for you to converse with them when they are less susceptible to the social norms of 'teenage' behaviour, meaning that there is sometimes space for them to open up in a way they may not feel they can with their parents, teachers or other significant adults in their lives. This can result in young people disclosing information to you about themselves or others at risk, so you have to be clear that you have a statutory duty to pass on any information about possible safeguarding issues. In such a position of both great trust and responsibility, it is important you do not make promises you may not be able to keep if a client asks you not to pass on information disclosed to you (especially if she or he is under 16, or has other capacity issues).

Concluding comments

Communicating with teenagers and adolescents can feel like a thankless task at times, with adults fearing they can say nothing right. However, it need not be such a source of mystery and/or trepidation, and can even be rewarding at times. An ability to empathise with their needs and concerns is vital, as well as to take time to consider the perspective they may have in your interactions with them. It always helps to have a good sense of humour and to not take yourself too seriously when working with them.

Competing narratives informing social identity

As discussed above, individual identities are formed according to social identity and self-categorisation principles. It is therefore worth considering related ways in which interpersonal communication within the clinical nursing environment may be influenced by implicit differences within and between some nursing and client cultures, around what is taken for granted but not usually openly expressed. On the basis of narrative research, Grant et al. (2015a) discussed how mental health staff and clients in their study storied the same events in mutually antagonistic ways on the basis of different narratives informing the motivations and experiences of the two groups. These authors argue that institutional mental health staff tend to privilege their storied explanations of events and the clients in their care as *the truth*, thus marginalising and dismissing the ways in which clients make sense of their, often distressing and abusive, experiences. This trend of 'culture-centrism' is played out in relationships between younger nurses and older people.

Communication between younger nurses and older persons

Some key issues of interpersonal communication between nurses and patients on the basis of group differences will be discussed later in this chapter. For the moment, consider the ways in which differences in speech and language, and overall communication, between, for example, young and older people, can often be marked. Younger nurses may assume that the way that they speak and dress is right and proper, and needs no justification, without considering the impact of all of this on people in their care. Although they may feel they're providing a good standard of care, they may fail to notice how their dress and conversational style excludes and disrespects patients. In this regard, as also stated in Chapter 7, the social-environmental communication context for nursing practice is crucial, and ethical and professional violations can easily occur because of the unquestioned dress and behaviour code of some employees.

Another stark example of nurses not paying sufficient attention to the person–situation context is in the use of what has been described as 'baby talk'. Over two decades ago, Ryan and Hamilton (1994) studied nurse–patient interactions with elderly nursing home residents. Some nurses demonstrated a lack of respect in their use of baby talk, and related voice tone and parental style. Nurses and volunteers using baby talk were rated less respectful and competent than their peers, and elderly recipients of baby talk were, understandably, less satisfied with interactions in which this occurred.

The use of baby talk and inappropriate clothing raises interesting questions about how many healthcare workers, including nurses, take for granted the cultural assumptions they have about themselves and the world and others within it, and, in related terms, their power relative to others. These questions alert us to the need to be mindful of how such assumptions develop, and also how they may be seriously compromised in the face of contemporary demands made on nurses to work sensitively with emerging groups and populations, such as trans communities (to be discussed in the next chapter). Such groups are rightly gaining the confidence to challenge the constraints imposed on them by normative assumptions.

Prejudice and schema development

From a cognitive developmental perspective, none of us are born with psychological maps or templates for understanding the world, other people or ourselves. These develop over time, mostly in childhood, as a result of our interactions in the world with significant others, particularly our parent or parents. Described as schemas, or core beliefs (Grant et al., 2008, 2010), they are necessary in enabling us to make sense of ourselves in interactions with others, and in changing life circumstances and situations.

Those of us fortunate enough to have good-enough parenting will develop schemas (see Chapter 2) which enable us to get by relatively reasonably successfully in the world, and with other people and ourselves. However, equally, because of abusive early life experiences, many of us will grow up with a core sense of ourselves as 'worthless', 'bad', 'useless' or something equally self-denigrating, which can lead to troubled relationships and sense of self throughout life.

Research and practice summary: Schemas as 'self-prejudice'

In her ground-breaking work on helping the kind of people described immediately above, Padesky (1991) explained how she helps her psychotherapy clients begin to consider how their deeply held negative schemas are a form of 'self-prejudice'. She does this by asking clients to bring to mind someone in their life who is deeply prejudiced. This prejudice may, for example, be directed towards certain groups of people because of their religious or sexual orientation. She then engages in a dialogue with them to help them review the ways in which such prejudices may be maintained through forms of selective information processing. This can include attending to information that confirms the 'truth' of the prejudice, while ignoring or discounting evidence that challenges it. Clients are then invited to consider the similarities between their own deeply held negative schemas and the prejudices and prejudiced people they have been discussing.

A strikingly ironic feature of deeply held prejudices, whether – in Padesky's terms – they are prejudices held against oneself or directed towards societal groups, is that they are often not experienced or regarded by the people who hold them as prejudices at all. Instead, they are considered to be right and proper, and common sense – a reflection of the world as it is, rather than a distortion of reality or a bigoted point of view. In order for people to begin to rid themselves of their prejudices, they have to begin to question them and see them as contingent (dependent on events and circumstances in their upbringing) rather than as absolutely true.

Nursing and dominant cultural beliefs

It may be helpful at this stage to consider the extent to which we all hold such culture-centric beliefs and assumptions about our life-worlds that remain taken for granted as 'just so' rather than potentially or actually problematic. Parfitt (1998) suggests that the majority of nursing care is delivered from the value position of nurses, and that this may therefore be based on their dominant cultural beliefs.

Narayanasamy and White (2005, p104) argue:

Ironically, the vast majority of indigenous healthcare workers have rarely, if ever, previously given consideration as to what their values and cultural beliefs are. Or how their values, beliefs and cultural traditions are acquired. Yet most assume, with equal measures of ignorance and arrogance, that their 'British' culture is the right way and that it is naturally superior to all other 'uncivilised or unsophisticated' cultures. Regrettably, those who possess this attitude will come into conflict with patients/clients who are not Anglicized or 'British'. That negative tension or cultural conflict, if not rapidly dispelled, will ultimately undermine the therapeutic relationship between patient and [nurse]; and therefore the quality of care will be compromised.

Padesky, and other cognitive psychotherapy writers (Hayes and Smith, 2005; Grant et al., 2008, 2010) argue that prejudices and other forms of deeply held belief are maintained through people engaging in speech and language, and related behaviour, that give form and substance to them. So, there are two interesting views of the world that may be useful to contemplate: in the first, the world is more or less separate from the language we use to describe it; in the second, the world is constituted or given shape, substance and reality by language.

Theory summary: The Sapir–Whorf hypothesis

That language defines the way a person behaves and thinks was proposed by Edward Sapir (1983) and his student and colleague Benjamin Whorf (1956). Both believed that language and the thoughts that we have are interwoven, and that all people are affected by the confines of their language. In short, they argued that humans are, in a sense, mental prisoners, unable to think freely because of the restrictions of their vocabularies.

An example of this idea is apparent in George Orwell's book *1984*, in which he discusses the use of a language he calls 'Newspeak', developed to change the way people thought about the government. The new vocabulary they were given was created to control their minds. Since they could not think of things not included in the vocabulary, they were, by default, linguistic zombies, imprisoned and deadened by the limits of their language. Sapir and Whorf coined the term *linguistic determinism* to capture the notion of ideas and creativity as the prisoners of vocabulary. If people indeed cannot think outside the confines of their language, the result of this process is many different world-views by speakers of different languages.

According to Sapir and Whorf, an idea complementary to linguistic determinism is 'linguistic relativity', which states that the differences in languages reflect the different views of people from different cultures. A key question emerging from this perspective is that if the world-view and behaviour of people are shaped by the structure of their language, and languages differ across cultures, then what are the threats to coherent cross-cultural communication and understanding in the modern world?

The Sapir–Whorf hypothesis indicates that absolute conceptual barrier-free communication seems unlikely. There is no question that the vocabulary of a specific language emphasises particular things, objects, events and experiences in a culture. For example, a society where horses are revered will have many words for horses and horse-related things because people in this society will talk about their horses a lot. Similarly, the Inuit people have many words for snow, the North Americans for cars and the Norwegians for fish. This does not necessarily mean that people from other cultures are incapable of perceiving the items that are described with such specific vocabulary, elsewhere. However, they are likely to nuance the meanings of these items through the perceptual lens related to their own specific cultures.

In criticism of the Sapir–Whorf hypothesis, if the English language was somehow keeping us from freedom of thought, we would all be trapped in the same cognitive path if we were English speakers. However, people from different cultural and ethnic backgrounds speak English as their main language, and even among siblings and close relatives, the understanding of certain words and what they mean varies. This is due to different environmental shaping factors to which people in the same family have been exposed, or expose themselves; to personal interests, friends and teachers, and perhaps to age and generational differences. If we were totally prisoners of our language, two people living in the same house with the same genetic make-up and speaking the same language should think and talk identically about issues, things, people and events. This is obviously not the case. That said, awareness of, and discussion around, the seminal contribution of the Sapir–Whorf hypothesis are important components of globalisation, communication and cultural education in the world today.

If the Sapir–Whorf hypothesis is still considered relatively useful, the degree to which we are all more or less 'trapped within' language in making sense of, and constructing, our worlds has fairly clear implications for nursing people from different cultures – and this includes cultures of ethnicity, race, sexuality, religion. For example, something that one cultural group takes for granted, in relation to healthcare and communication, may be alien and experienced as deeply strange by another group. This means that, as nurses, we must be very cautious about making rash cultural assumptions. It is easy, for example, to interact with people on the basis of a cultural stereotype which we think such people may immediately relate to and connect with, but which may be experienced as presumptuous and offensive by them.

Shifting friendship, family and cultural networks

It was argued above (Hogg and Vaughan, 2011), on the basis of social identity theory and self-categorisation theory, that social identity is experienced in relation to the primary reference group to which a person belongs, be it family and/or friends or colleagues. Within the space of a lifetime, an individual is likely to shift primary reference groups several, perhaps many, times and develop identities and related values and communication styles different from, and possibly in opposition to, their original reference groups.

Such shifts may appear radical in form. For example, the 1960s saw the emergence of Flower Power and Psychedelia. A decade later, the Punk and Anarcho Punk movements emerged, partly in reaction against the music, style, attitudes and forms of communication associated with Psychedelia, followed more recently by, among others, the Grunge and Goth movements. Such youth-, music- and style-related movements have been described as 'subcultures'. Subcultures exist in opposition, or run counter, to the dominant cultures within which they are embedded, while employing elements, materials and motifs from those cultures in novel ways to generate new cultural meanings (Hebdidge, 1979).

Within Britain, in addition to sub- and **countercultures**, shifting populations with their different health needs – for example, refugees – are currently moving within and between changing social contexts such as family structures and friendship networks. With regard to ethnic differences alone, this gives rise to a rich and complex multicultural picture, which has clear implications for the need for skilled interpersonal communication, and related awareness, among nurses.

Institutional racism

We now live in a country characterised, post-Brexit, by an increase in racist hate crime. At a healthcare organisational level, insensitive behaviour to people from different ethnic groups, whether it results from deeply held prejudices, ignorance or simply thoughtlessness, can often worsen already existing institutional racism.

Post-Brexit hate crime

On 17 November 2016, *The Independent* newspaper reported on the racial abuse experienced by EU nurses in the UK in the wake of the Brexit referendum result. Dame Julie

Case studies: Institutional racism

The Macpherson Report (1999) suggested that most of Britain's public institutions displayed institutional racism, defined as:

> *The collective failure of an organisation to provide an appropriate and professional service to people because of their colour, culture or ethnic origin. It can be seen or detected in processes, attitudes and behaviour which amount to discrimination through unwitting prejudice, ignorance, thoughtlessness and racist stereotyping which disadvantage minority ethnic people.*

(Macpherson of Cluny, 1999, p10)

Moore, Head of the University Hospitals Birmingham NHS Foundation Trust, reported to members of the House of Lords, who were holding an inquiry into NHS finances. She said that in the context of UK nursing shortages generally, and in her own Trust, EU nurses were looking to return to their country of origin because of such abuse. This phenomenon should be seen in the much larger national context of racial hate crimes in the UK, post-Brexit.

Retraumatisation in the mental health system

The word 'retraumatisation' simply means to be traumatised again, occurring when someone experiences something in the present that is reminiscent of a traumatic event in their past. The current event can evoke the emotional, physiological and behavioural responses associate with the original trauma, and powerlessness, all of which is frequently outside of the traumatised person's awareness. From a critical mental health perspective, institutional mental health treatment can often retraumatise because the fundamental operating principles of the international mental health system are based on coercion and control (Grant et al., 2015a). Sweeney et al. (2016) argue that mental health services are not only institutionally racist by recasting someone's understandable self-protective responses to being the victim of racism as individual pathology, but that this contributes to the accumulated historical and cultural trauma of racial and ethnic groups.

How do organisations frequently respond to such charges? Developing the propositions of psychoanalyst Sigmund Freud, Morgan (2006) argued that organisations, in terms of their collective worker mindset, are just like individuals in using unconscious protective measures to escape blame. Table 6.1 illustrates this argument in relation to institutional racism and related interpersonal communication difficulties.

According to Morgan (2006), organisational defence mechanisms, by definition, occur at an organisationally unconscious level. In relation to this, healthcare organisations have a tendency to socialise many of their members into a 'silent and tacit' agreement with the organisation's values and 'the way things are done around here'. Because of this, nurses may relatively rapidly forget the idealism they had when training in favour of buying into the kinds of organisational communication styles and difficulties described above.

Defence mechanism	Defence mechanism defined	Possible communication difficulties
Repression	Pushing unacceptable ideas and impulses into the unconscious	The possibility that abuse and communication neglect go on in our organisation is relegated to the organisational unconscious
Denial	Refusing to acknowledge a disturbing fact, feeling or memory	Presenting a public face of transculturalism while maintaining institutionally racist forms of communication and refusing to acknowledge this at an organisational level
Displacement	Shifting disturbing feelings aroused by one person on to a safer target	Maintaining that 'it is not our responsibility to display culturally sensitive forms of communication because we have not been trained in it'
Rationalisation	The creation of elaborate or unconvincing schemes of justification to disguise underlying motives and intentions	'Racism does not go on in our organisation. Difficulties in communication between nurses and ethnic minority patient groups are due to circumstances outside our control, including the failure of those patient groups to adapt sufficiently to take advantage of the care on offer'
Regression	Adopting behavioural patterns found satisfying and effective in childhood in order to reduce the effect of uncomfortable demands	Sending ethnic clients 'to Coventry', by avoiding them and avoiding talking with them
Splitting and idealisation	Inappropriately separating different elements of experience, and talking up the good aspects of a situation to avoid facing the bad ones	'We represent a centre of excellence in many aspects of our care and this has been acknowledged by feedback from many patients and articles in the local press'

Table 6.1　Organisational defence mechanisms (adapted from Grant et al., 2004)

The fallacy of individualism

A difficult but necessary question to pose is to what extent mainstream approaches to the dissemination of CIPS in nursing are culture-centric – embedded in cultural values.

A criticism of the widespread reliance on counselling models of interpersonal communication to inform interpersonal skills texts in nursing has been discussed earlier in this book. Developing this argument from the position of **culture-centrism**, it can be argued that Rogerian (see page 41) and related humanistic influences in CIPS in nursing betray the assumption of a taken-for-granted individualism.

From an individualistic standpoint, patients and nurses are assumed to have the innate psychological ability to find their own solutions to their problems, independent of the cultural, organisational, social or material constraining factors which give rise to such problems in the first place and maintain them. This assumption, which has a long legacy in some of the psychological therapies, has been contested vigorously from a critical psychological position (Smail, 2011). This challenges the overly simplistic idea that people can somehow rise above or effectively combat these constraining factors solely by their own efforts (see, for example, Grant and Leigh-Phippard, 2014).

Related to these critiques of individualism is the fact that environmental, organisational and cultural discourses (world-views) both shape and limit what can be done and said in any interpersonal exchange among nurses, between nurses and other healthcare workers, and between nurses and patients. Complementing the Sapir–Whorf hypothesis, discourse theory argues that none of us can avoid speaking from a particular discursive position (Speed, 2011). Put simply, there is no vocabulary or set of actions available to us, to talk about, and relate to, our worlds – professional and otherwise – which are free from the cultural meaning shaping that has already taken place before our entry into those worlds.

In spite of these difficulties with the individualistic stance, deriving from selective aspects of humanistic psychology generally (Whitton, 2003) and Rogerian counselling more specifically (Rogers, 2002), a simple, naive and overly optimistic picture of human interaction emerges. This is about two or more individuals interacting in a cultural and organisational–environmental vacuum.

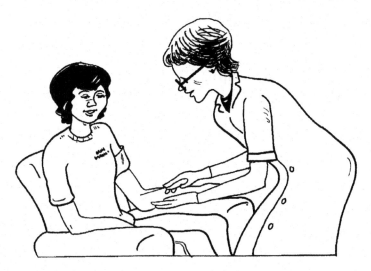

Figure 6.1 Simple picture of interaction

The humanistic picture of interaction in Figure 6.1 both contrasts with and masks a more challenging image of the nurse and patient interacting within multiple cultural and organisational environmental contexts, which have the power to shape and limit what can be said and done in the name of 'communication and interpersonal skills in nursing' (Figure 6.2).

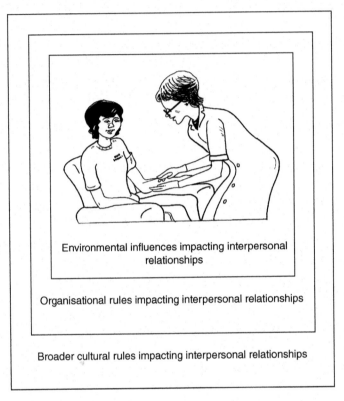

Environmental influences impacting interpersonal relationships

Organisational rules impacting interpersonal relationships

Broader cultural rules impacting interpersonal relationships

Figure 6.2   Complex picture of interaction

The individualist/counselling model of skilled communication

By placing sole responsibility for good CIPS on nurses, the organisation is let 'off the hook' for the kinds of environmental factors, described above, which work to undermine good communication. At a local cultural level, the unwritten rules, also described above, resulting from socialisation into organisations, impact on communication styles (Morgan, 2006). These rules, often held at unconscious levels, will affect the quantity and quality of communication between different professional groups and between health workers, including nurses, and patients.

Task, rather than holistic patient, workplace cultures will result in 'I–it' rather than 'I–thou' relationships (Buber, 1958). At a broader cultural level, institutional racism and sexism, cultural incompetence, and the prejudice that accompanies these problems, are often likely to influence the quality and quantity of nurse–patient interpersonal communication, but, unfortunately, remain under-acknowledged or denied.

Chapter summary

Different care settings may undermine the practice of safe and effective CIPS. Physical and social-environmental factors are very important for the practice of good communication in healthcare, in relation to communication both between and within groups, families and populations, and between younger and older people. 'Prejudice' and 'schema development', and their relation to language use, are key to understanding examples of poor CIPS in nursing. Institutional racism impacts negatively on communication and interpersonal exchanges in British nursing practice.

There is a variety of ways in which healthcare organisations defend themselves from accepting that they may be institutionally racist. The 'fallacy of individualism' in CIPS practice in British nursing masks the important role of environmental, organisational and broader cultural influences impacting upon such care.

Further reading

McDougall, T (2006) *Child and Adolescent Mental Health Nursing.* Oxford: Blackwell.

Rutter, M, Bishop, D, Pine, D, Scott, S, Stevenson, J, Taylor, E and Thapar, A (eds) (2010) *Rutter's Child and Adolesecent Psychiatry,* 5th edn. Oxford: Wiley-Blackwell.

Useful reading for working with children and adolescents.

Cioffi, J (2006) Culturally diverse patient–nurse interactions on acute care wards. *International Journal of Nursing Practice,* 12(6): 319–325.

Leininger, M (1997) Transcultural nursing research to nursing education and practice: 40 years. *Image Journal of Nursing Scholarship,* 29(4): 341–347.

One hundred culture-specific studies by Madeleine Leininger.

Harwood, J (2007) *Understanding Communication and Aging: Developing knowledge and awareness.* Thousand Oaks, CA: Sage Publications, Inc.

Engaging with these publications will help you become more familiar with research on transcultural nursing practices and on communication both between and with elderly clients.

Useful websites

www.bjmp.org/content/uncovering-face-racism-workplace

An interesting 2009 article on racism in healthcare and other work settings.

www.elderabuse.org.uk

A national resource on the issue of abuse of the elderly in care and nursing homes.

Chapter 7

Cultural diversity contexts of communication and interpersonal skills

Introduction

Society today is enriched by multicultural, ethnic and social, sexual, gender, religious and other forms of diversity. The focus of this chapter will be on the interpersonal and ethical contexts of interpersonal communication with people from diverse cultural backgrounds.

The chapter begins by exploring cultures, taking into account the range we experience in nursing and the differences that make up a society of diverse groups and identities. We will be investigating some of this terrain to gain a deeper understanding of the diversity (differences between people) and the potential for discrimination. We do so to trouble patterns of behaviour that can have a major detrimental effect on the lives of health service users, which are linked to discriminatory practices.

Some important issues of multicultural nursing will be explored, in relation to cultural awareness, cultural competence, and **transcultural** care. In examining diversity in a society that is made up of different groups, to which power, influence and opportunities are not always equally granted, we discuss the significance of race, gender, sexual orientation, age and disability.

The chapter concludes with a section that considers the ethical and moral consequences of communication and personal interactions.

Cultural diversity and difference

There is a constant danger that being different from the normative majority in any society will be equated with being inferior. Culture is a complex and multifaceted social phenomenon that affects our lives. To be an effective communicator with culturally diverse patients, a nurse has to be able to understand the different social structures and norms influencing values and behaviour in different societies. This knowledge enables nurses to engage with previously unfamiliar behaviour patterns and attitudes without dismissing or devaluing them. On a practical level, this requires interacting with service users and those close to them in appropriate, culturally congruent and acceptable ways.

Defining culture

Let us look at the concept and its meanings. The term 'culture' is often used to describe a very large social group based on a shared national origin, but it can mean patterns of behaviour and values of a group of people who participate in a particular shared identity. The term can also refer to a regional group, reflecting a collective sense of being through activities, traditions and language contained within a specific geographical area. In a narrower sense, in the context of the healthcare work settings you will find yourself in, an organisational culture implies a set of shared values and assumptions about 'the way things are done around here'.

As an inter-generational phenomenon, culture refers to a learned set of values, assumptions and behaviours transmitted through time. Generally speaking, this provides cultural members with a continuing and reliable sense of connectedness with others in their own community, while cultural 'outsiders' may be treated with mistrust and suspicion.

Culture affects every aspect of daily life: how we think, feel and behave, and make decisions and judgements. Such 'how we do and view things in our group' characteristics are in large measure acquired unconsciously in early childhood. We are born into culture which plays a large part in shaping our social thinking styles (Augoustinos et al., 2014). That said, it is equally true that we do not have to regard our cultural identity as fixed and determined. A trawl through the writings of social philosophers and theorists such as Michel Foucault and Judith Butler helps us better understand how we can and do resist, mutate, nuance, co-shape, and re-invent our personal, relational and community cultural identities.

Activity 7.1   Reflection

- To appreciate how culture is learned, identify and describe one custom or tradition in your own family or community group. Ask your parent, grandparent or an elder where the custom originated. Has the custom or tradition changed over the years and can your relative or elder tell you why?
- Can you also think of a custom that you have adopted, but that is relatively new in your family or social group? Can you trace why this has happened, and the source of this custom?

Hint: This activity might help you understand how some cultures become assimilated into the mainstream, or not, and relates to the following topics of multiculturalism and acculturation.

'Multiculturalism' is the term used to describe a heterogeneous society in which many diverse cultural groups geographically coexist and constantly mutate. All groups will share general characteristics, while some characteristics will be unique to particular groups within the larger multicultural whole. However, society is becoming increasingly global due to changes in demographics, the internet and an interdependent world economy. The movement towards shared cultural characteristics and mores, increased interracial marriage or partnership relationships between communities, corresponds to the transmission of traditional and new cultural behaviours and beliefs via media and the internet. Conversely, these very factors can also provoke culturally conservative reactions. Some groups invest great energy in ongoing attempts to retain their cultural differences, to ward off change and a feared dilution of their cultural beliefs in the face of perceptions of global cultural homogenisation and colonisation.

Given the above, 'cultural diversity' is a blanket term used to understand current and emerging dynamic differences among cultural groups in society. Cultural diversity can be seen across nationality, ethnic origin, age, gender, sexuality, lifestyle, values, educational background, geographic location, economic status, language, politics and religion. There can also be sub-diversity within what appear to be homogeneous societal groups, such as in health and social care occupational work cultures settings. Physicians, social workers, healthcare assistants, nurses, administrators, porters and physiotherapists each have their own cultural and sub-cultural identities, rituals and practices. These can affect decisions, the allocation of tasks, and how values are shared and contested within these groups, in dynamic and constantly shifting ways. In light of this, conflict within and between groups is inevitable, but should not always be regarded as destructive.

Case study: The mental health specialist

Alexandra comes from a mental health nursing background, has a Master's degree in cognitive behavioural psychotherapy (CBP), and is accredited as a CBP psychotherapist, supervisor and teacher with the British Association of Behavioural and Cognitive Psychotherapies. Since coming into post, she has occasionally received requests from a mental health day hospital in her area to provide therapy for clients. When these requests were first made, she found the system of referral was mostly too informal for her liking, to the extent that day hospital clients often had no idea they were being referred or why referral was necessary in the first place. Moreover, she soon discov- the day hospital nursing staff making the requests had a poor knowledge of onship between psychological disorders and appropriate interventions. On ion, this resulted in a client being referred for 'exposure therapy' because arent 'phobia of getting on buses' near his home. On assessment of this cli- ndra found that his problem was not one of phobic anxiety. It was because a group of local thugs, with a vendetta against his family, knew he frequently used these buses and were out to get him.

Alexandra identified cultural differences between the generic mental health nursing service and herself around the communication involved in good 'referral etiquette' (Grant, 2010d), and knowledge of psychopathology and evidence-based psychotherapy. She resolved to address these through a series of teaching workshops for day hospital staff.

'**Cultural relativism**' refers to the understanding that cultures are not intrinsically inferior or superior to one another. Furthermore, individuals within cultures will not only ascribe different levels of meaning and importance to cultural beliefs and behaviours, but will violate and mutate them in myriad ways. This means that someone who appears to belong to a culture may not follow all of its practices, and this applies equally to nursing. Consequently, customs, attitudes, rituals and beliefs have to be understood according to the individual needs and standpoint of each patient.

The antonym to cultural relativism is '**ethnocentrism**', a term which refers to people who believe that their nation, culture or imagined ethnic group is superior to others. There are several examples of this in history; for example Hitler and the Nazis, and white supremacists in the USA. To be proud of one's identified culture is of course reasonable, but if this is taken to extremes cultural oppression is the outcome, as evidenced by the increase in hate crimes against those not perceived to 'belong' in the UK, in the wake of the Brexit referendum.

'**Discrimination**' is an aspect of ethnocentrism that refers to the marginalisation of some societal groups, such as the physically or learning disabled, people engaged with mental health services, those in poverty, the homeless, persons with HIV, or refugees. When access to healthcare is increasingly inhibited through discrimination in healthcare provision, this constitutes an insidious act of **ethnocentricity**.

Theory summary: Measuring prejudice and discrimination

Gordon Allport (1954) devised a scale of prejudice and discrimination, and it is useful to consider how individuals might slowly slide down the scale. Knowledge of this scale might lead to an awareness of seemingly trivial actions which, if unchecked, might lead to serious consequences, especially if they are accompanied by 'thoughtlessness' (see Minnich, 2017, and Chapters 10 and 11 of this book).

(Continued)

(Continued)

The scale is:

1. **Antilocution** includes hate speech. An 'in group' freely discusses negative images of an 'out group', for example, 'old people are demented' or 'schizos are dangerous'.
2. **Avoidance** where the 'in group' actively isolates or avoids the 'out group'. Consider the extent we do this to old people.
3. **Discrimination** involving the denial of opportunities and services to the 'out group'.
4. **Physical attack** involving assault or abuse, for example, in care environments. The 'out group's' property may also be destroyed or stolen.
5. **Extermination** – the removal or even killing of members of the 'out group'.

Although extreme examples can be thought of, if we identify people with learning disabilities or frail older people, is there a possibility that less extreme stages of prejudice exist currently?

Theory summary: Ethnocentrism

The process of socialisation into the occupation of nursing carries with it the need to internalise its dominant cultural values. Because of this, nursing is not culture-free, but is embedded in shifting cultural values that pervade all aspects of care, practice and knowledge, including CIPS. If this is neither acknowledged nor understood, nurses can be charged with being guilty of gross, unacknowledged ethnocentrism. Two decades ago, Parfitt (1998, p52) asserted: *Nurses who hold ethnocentric views will be unable to interpret their patients' behaviour appropriately as they will judge it according to the norms of their own behaviour.*

The extent to which ethnocentric cultural values still prevail in the NHS is a crucial issue. Parfitt saw the NHS as *reflecting the cultural norm of not only the white majority but the middle class white majority.* To the extent that this state of affairs still exists, privileged white British values and assumptions are taken as 'common sense' and 'right and proper', against which ethnic and cultural minorities are located and labelled as 'the other'. This has obvious implications for the prevalence of discrimination, institutional racism and witting or unwitting prejudice among healthcare workers.

Sawley (2001) highlighted racist incidents in nursing and healthcare. These included black colleagues being referred to in derogatory terms; white relatives being allowed to use the patients' toilets with Asian relatives barred; white staff making racist remarks against Asians; and Asian patients not permitted to have large numbers of visitors, while white patients were not subjected to such controls. These practices are clearly reflective of discrimination in the form of racist prejudice in the wider societal context, which Figure 7.1 may help illustrate.

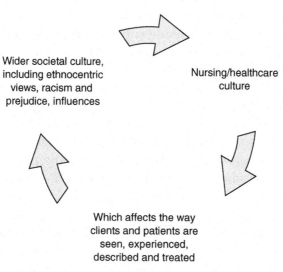

Wider societal culture, including ethnocentric views, racism and prejudice, influences

Nursing/healthcare culture

Which affects the way clients and patients are seen, experienced, described and treated

Figure 7.1　Racist prejudice in the wider societal context

Cultural competence

Cultural competence refers to an ability to interact effectively with people of different cultures. It is comprised of four components:

- awareness of one's own cultural world-view;
- attitude towards cultural differences;
- knowledge of different cultural practices and world-views;
- cross-cultural skills.

Developing cultural competence results in an ability to understand, communicate with, and effectively interact with people across cultures – in short, to be culturally sensitive.

Anderson et al. (2007) explored the principles of involving the community to strengthen cultural competence in nurse education, practice and research in order to reduce the health disparities in communities. Their findings included the importance of reducing and levelling differences in power between practitioners and the community. It also clearly emerged that communication and relationships between healthcare workers and community members have to be culturally appropriate, and that it was crucially important to work hard to develop trust. Overall, reflecting the importance of the 'I–thou' rather than the 'I–it' relationship discussed in Chapters 1 and 6, it was considered essential that interventions were done 'with' rather than 'to' people.

In a complementary argument, focusing on the experience of pain, Lovering (2006) asserted that patients and health professionals bring their own cultural attitudes to interpret and talk about patients' pain experience, with the health professionals' knowledge and attitudes dominating. Lovering suggested that this situation could be improved through learning about the differing cultural attitudes towards pain held by both cultural groups and health staff. The rationale for this was that, through such learning, staff and patients from differing cultural groups can work with each other as opposed to the former 'doing to' the latter.

Cioffi (2006) conducted qualitative research in Australia. This explored experiences of interaction between nurses and minority ethnic patients. Nurses and patients from Asian or Middle Eastern Islamic backgrounds were interviewed individually about perceptions of the care provided. Issues identified were tensions arising from the Islamic groups' fear of discrimination, the requirements of visiting relatives, nurses' gender, perceived cultural differences and problems of communication and information exchange.

A decade earlier, Gerrish et al. (1996) recommended ways in which transcultural healthcare might be transmitted. According to these authors, it is crucial that nurses develop cultural sensitivity. In this context, the nurse should assume the role of tourist (with the good manners that go with that role), practise reflexive honesty (including the ways in which power may be distributed in favour of the health practitioner), explore the cultural meanings of ethnicity, strive for good intercultural communication and work to eradicate institutional and all other forms of racism.

Culture without cultural awareness

In the context of ethnocentricity, culture and institutional racism, in line with prejudice more generally, it is ironic that members of dominant cultures are likely to remain unaware that they have a specific culture. In terms of their social identity, what they regard as normal and universal assumptions, beliefs and behaviours are only 'normal' relative to their class, time and social groups. In contrast, those who have grown up as minority ethnic group members, or who have lived outside or away from their own society, are more likely to be acutely aware of the influence of culture as a result of being cultural 'outsiders'.

Transcultural nursing

As discussed in Chapter 1, 'caring' needs to be appraised through a transcultural lens (Leininger, 1997). In related terms, the quest for 'self-awareness' needs to be broadened to subjecting oneself to challenges to one's assumptions (Gerrish et al., 1996), because without the opportunities for self-awareness development in this transcultural sense, healthcare workers are likely to remain insensitive to other cultural values. This speaks to relational ethics (see Chapter 1) in that the imposition of one's own values on others can be offensive and unprofessional (MacNaught, 1994; Baxter, 2000).

Alec Grant, the first author of this book trained as a student mental health nurse in the early 1970s. He witnessed several examples of cultural insensitivity through British nurses renaming their ethnically different colleagues with British names. For example, a male colleague from the Republic of the Philippines, whose first name was difficult to pronounce, became 'Fred'. Less understandably, a Danish nurse named 'Elsa' was renamed 'Elsie'.

Fortunately, the awareness of the need for cultural sensitivity has increased since the 1970s. However, Narayanasamy and White (2005) argued that healthcare services should be more culturally responsive since, at that time, the cultural healthcare needs of ethnic minority groups were still not adequately met. It seems likely that there is still a failure of multicultural education, structures and policies, and transcultural health-care practice (Gerrish et al., 1996) to be adequately realised. The need for nurses to work at developing better standards of transcultural nursing care never ends.

Such care should extend to sensitivity towards shared social identities (Robb and Douglas, 2004) of people in groups sharing common experiences and needs. Among other factors, these are characterised by ethnicity, gender, disability, age and sexuality, all of which structure people's everyday experiences, including being in receipt of healthcare. Unfortunately, social identity can be used to discriminate against people, as 'other' or 'different', against a supposed 'norm'.

Activity 7.2   Critical thinking

A Bangladeshi woman is admitted to hospital for two weeks for an operation. Afterwards, she reports that she felt stupid during her stay in hospital because of her lack of English. 'Two nurses neglected me. I'm not sure if it was because of the colour of my skin or because of a language barrier. I'm still not sure what operation I had, and why.'

In small groups, discuss these questions.

- What is the nature of the communication problem experienced by the woman?
- Whose problem is it?
- What are the consequences for the speaker?

Hint: This activity should help you rehearse some of the transcultural nursing issues you may encounter as a student nurse and post-qualifying.

The questions raised in Activity 7.2 demonstrate the complexities of the issues, rather than easy answers. The answers you came up with will relate to your own cultural understanding of the nature of 'difference', how it is produced and how it should be responded to. For example, one possible answer is that the 'cause' of the problem was the woman's poor command of spoken English coupled with her lack of confidence, either because of her language difficulties or her cultural background.

However, equally, it could be argued that the communication problem arose because of the hospital's failure to address indirect and direct discrimination in its practices. Indirect discrimination was apparent in the failure to take account of the diverse needs of patients by, for example, failing to ensure the provision of bilingual workers or interpreters available for the main community languages in the area. Direct discrimination was apparent in how the two nurses ignored the woman.

The point is that nurses, like all humans, understand 'difference' differently. Related to social cognition-based discussions in this book on labelling, 'cognitive miserliness' (see Chapter 3) and prejudices, health workers often associate 'difference' with the membership of particular groups. These groups are perceived to have specific qualities, ways of communicating and communication needs.

Focusing on diversity

Diversity is about us as individual beings. As discussed earlier, society is made up of a variety of groups and in this section we will explore some of those groups from a sociological perspective, around socio-economic position, race and culture, gender, sexual orientation, age and disability.

Socio-economic position

An individual's socio-economic position is closely linked to factors such as income, wealth and social status. The Office of National Statistics (ONS) uses a classification system to gather data on the population, constructed around the UK economy, population and society at national, regional and local levels. According to Rose and Pevalin (2005), the first detailed classification was designed in 1928 and was intended to identify differences in economic distribution and status. Classification by socio-economic group was introduced in 1951 and aimed to categorise people according to their occupations and economic status. The ongoing development of these classification systems over the decades since their inception reflects the increasing complexity of the structure of our society. Other work relating to discussions on inequalities in health includes the Great British Class Survey (Savage et al., 2013) and Guy Standing's (2014) exposition on 'The Precariat'.

Politically and sociologically, class differentials have been the subject of much debate and continue to be used to delineate social divisions in society, the distribution of wealth and various forms of inequality relative to the rest of the world (Wilkinson and Pickett, 2010; Scambler, 2012). The gap in the share of income between the richest and the poorest has increased globally. Added to this are economic changes that have affected society, such as the decrease in traditional working-class employment in the manufacturing industry and the increase in service industries.

Nurses are expected to work fairly with people from all aspects of life, so when communicating with persons from different socio-economic backgrounds it is important not to make assumptions based upon class and other cultural stereotypes. People move from one group to another, as a result of a variety of circumstances. There is a danger that collusion can occur between similar groups and issues can be overlooked, for example middle-class health visitors overlooking child abuse in middle-class families. Nurses also need to be wary of other stereotyping assumptions, such as that the most educated need less explanation of their health problems and treatment, while those with less education need more, or that people with mental health problems do not need to be routinely informed about the short- and long-term side-effects of their prescribed medications.

Race and culture

The UK has a population that is composed of a wide variety of cultures, religions and languages. Over 300 different languages are currently spoken in London schools. While there are differing concentrations of multiculturalism throughout its four countries, the UK is no longer a white homogeneous nation. To think so is to devalue the minority cultures within our society and disregard crucial aspects of people's lives and values. This can lead to racist attitudes and discrimination, and can thus act as a barrier to good practice in healthcare. Communication and interpersonal interactions need to be ethnically sensitive and anti-racist. Assumptions, for example on skin colour determining biological differences, have the potential to be used as arguments for the destructive mythology of racial inferiority. Taking the time to understand cultural and ethnic beliefs and practices is needed, as well as listening to the stories of friends and colleagues who have been harassed or abused.

Gender

From a normative perspective (Zeeman et al., 2014b), there is an acknowledgement of recognisable differences between men and women in most societies, and a corresponding male/female divide that has various codes and expectations of behaviour and responses in social interaction. From this perspective, by the age of two, infants can recognise the differences through hair and clothes, aided by significant gender stereotyping prevalent in most societies. The extent to which gender differences are innate or learned is, however, the subject of debate. In current times, the concept of 'gender fluidity' troubles traditional assumptions of natural gender binaries. The apparently straightforward binary divide between 'male' and 'female' is challenged by contemporary theoretical and empirical work on health and healthcare, and in line with theorists such as Judith Butler, a more contemporary view is that gender is something we 'do' rather than something we 'are' (Zeeman et al., 2014b). In contrast, 'cisnormativity' refers to the assumption that most 'normal' people self-identify with their biological appearance. However, the contemporary plural terms 'masculinities' and 'femininities' give the lie to this assumption.

That said, there continues to be a palpable unequal distribution of power and life chances between genders. In response to this, nurses need to be constantly sensitive to how women are treated in healthcare settings to ensure that their expressed needs and difficulties are not overlooked and are treated with respect. In this regard, it is important to ensure that women's problems are *discussed in women's terms*, and that stereotypical gender expectations and perceptions are challenged if they are without evidence or foundation. A contemporary example of this is in the area of stalking, where the reported experiences of women who have been subjected to this are often trivialised, ignored, or put down to hysterical over-reaction, by health and social care workers, and by the legal and police services (Taylor et al., 2018).

Men can also experience problems, when, as a result of cultural stereotyping, certain responses are expected from them around how they think, feel and act. This is particularly evident at times of bereavement, and in relation to suicide (Grant et al., 2013). In the light of these examples, when men and women interact within a context of gender-based cultural stereotyping, barriers to communication and interpersonal relationships can undermine effective assessment and health interventions. This can exacerbate or reinforce the pre-existing problems of users of health and social care (for example, in areas such as low self-esteem) and close down helpful dialogue about the issues and problems being presented.

Sexual orientation

From the perspective that sexuality is purely, or primarily, a biological phenomenon, and heterosexuality natural and normal, homosexuality is inevitably defined as unnatural and abnormal. This heteronormative view discriminates against many members of society. If the concept of sexuality is based on heteronormative assumptions, implicitly limited to the biological argument, this increases the likelihood of misunderstandings, prejudice and discrimination occurring in health and mental health care settings (Grant et al., 2016; Zeeman et al., 2014b).

It has to be acknowledged that gay and lesbian relationships are accepted in some cultures but not in others, where same-sex couples could face severe punishment or death. This creates an additional dilemma for health professionals. On the one hand, they should be prepared to help persons regardless of their sexual orientation. On the other, they will also need to take into account the beliefs of persons in their care who may not accept homosexuality, through reasons of faith or culture. Nurses' own cultural beliefs could be challenged in such circumstances. As with other diverse groups, respect, fairness and dignity are important features of working in a professional and non-judgemental manner, and are the precepts to be guided by in these encounters in the healthcare context.

Communication with members of the trans communities

It is important to be aware that 'gender identity' is separate from sexual orientation. Sexual orientation refers to the gender or genders that someone is sexually attracted to, whereas gender identity refers to the ways in which a person describes how they experience themselves in relation to a complex of issues around their embodiment and individual, relational and cultural lived-experiences.

The word 'trans' is an umbrella term, used to describe people whose sex/gender diverges in some ways from the sex/gender assigned to them at birth, and to transgendered men and women who seek treatment and surgical interventions to modify their bodies. However it is also used to refer to people who live outside of dominant gender norms without seeking surgical interventions. Some trans people identify as heterosexual, some as LGBQUI (lesbian, gay, bisexual, queer, undecided or intersex), whereas others may refuse sexual and/or gender categorisation or language which attempts to describe or define this. The trans communities therefore include the following groups (note that this is not an exhaustive or definitive list):

Transgender, transsexual, genderqueer, intersex, non-binary, bi-gender, genderfluid, cross-dresser, trans men, trans women, and agender.

Activity 7.3   Critical thinking

Individually, explore the meanings of all of the above terms, in relation to 'cisgender', 'heteronormativity' and 'homonormativity'.

Then in groups, discuss the implications emerging for the professional relationships between nurses and those who would regard themselves as members of the trans communities, which will include clients, patients, users, survivors, relatives and other nurses and healthcare staff, around:

- The choice of personal pronouns that trans individuals might want to be represented by, verbally and in writing (e.g. 'he', 'she', 'they').
- The tensions that nurses might find themselves in with regard to the above, between medico-legal practices and constraints and the freedom of self-representation at an individual level.

Now read and discuss the following two papers in small groups:

(Continued)

(Continued)

Aramburu Alegria, C (2011) Transgender identity and health care: implications for psychosocial and physical evaluation. *Journal of the American Academy of Nurse Practitioners*, 23: 175–182.

Grant, A, Naish, J and Zeeman, L (2016) Depathologising sexualities in mental health services. *Mental Health Practice*, 19(7): 26–31.

Hint: Engaging in all of these activities will help you around the need to exercise sensitivity in interpersonal relationships with these groups of people.

To summarise, we live in times where sexuality does not necessarily coincide with gender, where neither sexuality nor gender are always clear categories for capturing people's experiences and behaviour, and thus where traditional binaries for describing people – 'man'/'woman', heterosexual'/'homosexual' – are often and arguably increasingly regarded as inadequate and sometimes inappropriate in the face of gender and sexual fluidity. Prosser (2013, p34), for example, recently described 'trans' as an 'incessant destabilising movement between sexual and gender identities', signalling one of the overall aims and functions of Queer scholarship in disrupting and troubling binaried identities (Zeeman et al., 2014a, 2014b).

In her generally important resource for practice, Arambura Alegria (2011, p179) argued that it is important to address 'transgender persons in a gender-appropriate manner'. She went on to argue on the basis of this assertion that persons who have transitioned from male to female should be addressed as women and, conversely, persons who have transitioned from female to male should be addressed as men.

This may indeed seem, and often be, an appropriate courtesy strategy for nurses to adopt. However, Alegria's advice may be regarded as presumptuous and inappropriate by some transgendered patients, clients, service users or mental health survivors. This is because of the fluidity of identity and related self-referential terms highlighted in both the list of possible categories and the Queer scholarship described above. Thus, tact, sensitivity and checking out with people on the use of personal pronouns and gender-related descriptive language are crucial first steps in establishing good interpersonal relationships in these cultural contexts.

Age

Ageism is a term generally applied to discrimination against older persons, although it can be applied to children. When applied to older persons it can be characterised by a number of factors.

- *Marginalisation* – older people and their needs are rarely seen as a priority or a central concern.

- *Dehumanisation* – older people are represented as 'over the hill' and of little use to society.
- *Infantalisation* – older people tend to be treated like children, for example by using first names or nicknames, without asking the person if this is acceptable, or through the use of 'baby talk'.

The phenomenon of social ageing, or how we behave in social encounters towards each other, and our understanding of the differences between ourselves and others as we age or change are thought to be achieved through communication. Our own age, and the ages of those with whom we interact, shape our responses, behaviours and expectations. Therefore, we take the target of our responses into consideration and frame them accordingly. So, for example, a reward for a child would be, 'You're a clever little person', for an adolescent, 'You have really grown up' and for an older person it could be, 'I find your ideas very interesting'. Adapting to make the appropriate response is how we can work towards reducing ageism and guard against being patronising.

Reaction times, speech recognition and the capacity for information processing slow down with ageing; however, this happens at a different rate for different individuals. Older people have often had years of experience in dealing with people from different backgrounds and in different situations, and have gained a wealth of language to use in these contexts. Regrettably, the negative stereotyping of older people frequently results in nurses using secondary baby talk, 'elderspeak' and patronising talk with them. This is often the result of intentions to be helpful, such as slowing down or simplification of messages and clarification exercises, for example raising the volume of the voice, deliberate articulation and diminutives such as 'dear' or 'love'. However, as well as being demeaning, this has a negative effect on the self-identity of elderly people and can reinforce their sense of loss of control and dependency.

Theory Summary: Gerotranscendence

Tornstam (1997) discussed the idea of 'gerotranscendence', which suggests that growing old is part of normal development which can result in us progressing towards being more mature and wise. It is a positive view of ageing. If this is the case, the nurse should understand that age is not necessarily a negative experience and should accept that older people indeed have a degree of understanding about life that brings positive benefits. This theory, Tornstam suggests, is a counter to 'disengagement theory', in that the older person engages in new perspectives and understandings rather than withdrawing, or disengaging, from society.

See: **Tornstam, L** (1997) Gerotranscendence in a broad cross sectional perspective. *Journal of Aging and Identity*, 2(1): 17–36.

Nurses can think about pitching their responses at the appropriate level, having first assessed the ability (rather than chronological age) of the other person.

It may also be useful for nurses to critique assumptions about older people disengaging from society and instead think of them as having far more positive views about themselves and their life. See, for example, Tornstam's (1997) work on the theory of gerotranscendence.

Communicating with people who have dementia

Dementia is a huge topic area worthy of a book on its own. A good starting point though is Tom Kitwood's (1997) concepts of 'person-centred care', 'malignant social psychology' and 'positive person work' (Mitchell and Agnelli, 2015). The first stage is accepting the *personhood* of those you work with, which involves recognition, respect and trust. This might sound obvious but the fact that it has to be stated might indicate that the personhood of people with dementia has not always been established in our interpersonal relationships.

The second stage is considering and understanding 'malignant social psychology' (MSP). This refers to a wide range of behaviours which undermine personhood and which often arises through lack of education rather than malicious intent. Kitwood described malignancies such as *Treachery* – deceiving the person to distract or manipulate, *Mockery* – making fun or joking at their expense (which could form part of Allport's (1954) first stage of discrimination – antilocution) and *Objectification* – treating the person as an object, for example during the activity of living of personal hygiene, washing and dressing.

Then you need to learn 'positive person work' to address MSP. Kitwood identified concepts such as *Recognition* – recognising people by name, acknowledging they have unique thoughts, feelings and preferences, so calling them by a preferred name; *Play* – providing appropriate activity and enablement of self-expression and *Validation* – accepting the reality of another even if it is the results of hallucination or misperceptions.

Disability

Disability is often viewed as a physical problem that stands in the way of normal social functioning. An alternative view is that cultural attitudes to disability are potentially more disabling than the impairment itself. For example, it is not the use of a wheelchair that bars access to buildings; it is the lack of disabled access and a ramp that causes the disability. The social model of disability draws attention to the tendency for disabled people to be discriminated against, marginalised, dehumanised, patronised, with a focus more on their limitations rather than their potentials and capabilities.

Here are some suggestions for improving your CIPS skills when working with people with disabilities:

- Avoid negative terms and terms that define the person as disabled, such as 'the disabled man' or 'the handicapped child'.
- Instead, say 'person with a disability', always emphasising the person rather than the disability. Avoid describing the person with a disability as 'abnormal'; when you define people without disabilities as 'normal', you say, in effect, that the person with the disability isn't normal.
- Treat assistive devices such as wheelchairs, canes, walkers or crutches as the personal property of the user. Don't move these out of your way; they're for the convenience of the person with the disability. Avoid leaning on a person's wheelchair – it is similar to leaning on the person.
- Shake hands with the person with the disability if you shake hands with others in the group. Don't avoid shaking hands because the individual's hand is disfigured or misshapen, for example.
- Avoid talking about the person with a disability in the third person. For example, avoid saying 'Doesn't he get around beautifully with the new crutches?' Direct your comments to the individual.
- Don't assume that people who have a disability are intellectually impaired. Slurred speech, such as may occur with cerebral palsy or cleft palate, should never be taken as indicating a low-level intellect. Be especially careful not to talk down to people.
- When you're unsure how to act, ask. For example, if you're not sure if you should offer walking assistance, say 'Would you like me to help you into the dining room?' And, more importantly, accept the person's response. If he or she says no, that means no! So don't insist.
- Maintain similar eye level. If the person is in a wheelchair, for example, it might be helpful for you to sit down or kneel down to maintain the same eye level.

Broader ethical and moral considerations

Because there are consequences of interpersonal communication, whether deliberate or unintentional, there are also broader ethical considerations to take into account. Each communication situation has a moral dimension of rightness and wrongness, where the expectation is that communication will be honest, decent, just and appropriate. These moral principles are often expected and implicit in interactions. There is an expectation that nurses will respect individuals and act within the NMC *Code of Professional Conduct*, which embodies these principles. Within a cultural context, these have to be considered and interpreted according to the respective value systems of each culture.

A first step towards making decisions that take account of cultural variability is to understand the ways in which culture influences how health and illness are understood by the members of a cultural group or community sharing the same values. The cultural interpretation of health and illness is mediated by values and perceptions which are the product of the combination of traditions, lived experiences and the knowledges sanctioned by particular cultures. Values and perceptions are often derived from the notion of health as a resource, in terms of how this features in daily lives and affects the productivity, effectiveness, significance and status of people in cultural communities.

The dominant framework for understanding the cause and treatment of ill health in the Western world is the **biomedical model**. This conceptualises illness in terms of bodily malfunction requiring treatment cure, often through technical and pharmacological means. The biomedical model is based upon the broader scientific notion of progress resulting from quantitative-experimental research. The assumption is that the model provides a truthful account of reality when compared to more primitive forms of healing and curing practices, which are not empirically based and hence irrational.

While the biomedical model has clear and obvious value for healthcare generally, its application and consequences are not always culturally sensitive or beyond scientific reproach. In the context of critical mental health, for example, the diagnostic categories for understanding extremes of human misery are scientifically flawed. These categories lack acceptable levels of validity and reliability, and are Western culture-centric. They are often used to categorise mental health service users on the basis of social and ethnocentric, rather than sound and convincing biomedical diagnostic, judgements (Grant, 2015; Smith and Grant, 2016).

Case study: A complex interaction of responses

Alisha is 42 years old and works as a cleaner in an office building in a large UK city. She came to the UK from West Bengal, India, 22 years ago as a young bride. She barely makes a living and depends upon her work to supplement her husband's wages and support her family of five children, two of whom are adults but unemployed and living at home. In discussing her health, Alisha reveals a complex interaction of responses. If she considers the illness to be very serious she will as a last resort go to the local hospital, even though she knows she will have to wait a long time to be seen and it will be difficult to explain to the nurses and doctors why she is there, because her English is limited. For persistent fevers in her children she will go to the local allopathic doctor (using remedies whose effects differ from those produced by the disease), even though there will be high fees to pay, because she will not have to wait. In other instances, she may visit the homeopathic doctor, who is more affordable. She will also visit the kobiraj (the Ayurvedic practitioner). Finally, while Alisha knows that allopathic medicine offers relief, she equally knows it will not cure. For this to happen, Alisha believes the underlying causes have to be dealt with and these are connected to divine forces. To solve this problem, Alisha makes offerings at the temple of the goddess Kali so that she will be appeased.

This case study gives an example of the centrality of culture to perceptions of health and illness. It also illuminates the different resources and organisational structures to which individuals may resort for solutions to health problems. The notion of a divine basis for health, and models other than the biomedical utilised by Alisha to understand the cause and cure of illness, indicate a cultural terrain where the meanings of health and illness are subject to negotiation and contestation. Alisha's story involves shifting from one form of treatment to another depending on what is perceived as the nature of the illness, the location of the person in the family structure and its wider culture, and the price and time it takes to receive treatment and transport. These options are interwoven into a complex web of meaning involving hierarchies and resources. This calls for ethical decision making on the part of the nurse, deploying communication skills to enable a deeper understanding of cultural values and issues.

Chapter summary

In this chapter we have considered the extent to which the UK population is changing and the need for increased understanding and awareness of multicultural needs in healthcare. We have explored the ways in which the culture concept can be understood, and have considered the diverse population needs of groups in society in relation to social categories, race and culture, gender, sexual orientation, age and disability. Finally, we looked at some of the broader ethical and moral dimensions of communication and interpersonal relationships impacting on our culturally diverse worlds.

Further reading

Dutte, MJ (2008) *Communicating Health: A culture-centred approach.* Cambridge: Polity Press.
This book explores health communication from the perspective of culture.

Clarke, V, Ellis, SJ, Peel, E and Riggs, DW (2010) *Lesbian, Gay, Bisexual, Trans and Queer Psychology: An introduction.* Cambridge: Cambridge University Press.

Prosser, J (2013) Judith Butler: queer feminism, transgender, and the transubstantiation of sex. In: Hall, DE, Jagose, A, with Bebell, A and Potter, S (eds) *The Routledge Queer Studies Reader.* London and New York: Routledge.

Zeeman, L, Aranda, K and Grant, A (2014) *Queering Health: Critical challenges to normative health and healthcare.* Ross-on-Wye: PCCS Books.

These three books will help you explore in greater depth the interpersonal and communication implications related to working with trans populations, and understanding health and healthcare needs in terms of *difference*, and individual and cultural self-determination rather than *pathology*.

Useful websites

www.ons.gov.uk/ons/taxonomy/index.html?nscl=International+Migration

For information on immigration and migration.

swhr.org

The website for the Society for Women's Health Research.

www.lgbtnetwork.org

The website of the LGBT network.

www.clareproject.org.uk/home/support/support-resources

The Clare Project booklet *So, Someone You Know is Transgender, Questions and Answers for Family, Friends and Colleagues* is available on this website.

Chapter 8   Beyond technique

Chapter aims

After reading this chapter, in relation to the increasingly skilled practice of CIPS, you should be able to:

- understand the differences between **professional artistry** and **technical rationality** at theoretical and applied levels;
- describe what is meant by **critical reflexivity**;
- outline the place of critical reflexivity in the tensions between professional artistry and technical rationality in nursing;
- understand the significance of these tensions in the development of compassion in organisations;
- describe the place and significance of critical reflexivity in healthcare organisational development.

Introduction

Having got this far in your reading of the book, and as a bridge to the chapters that follow, we now want to take you in this chapter to a place 'beyond technique'. This place is not explicitly linked to NMC competencies or Essential Skills Clusters because it speaks to issues that are either broader, deeper and arguably more profound, or simply more human, than can be adequately captured in contemporary nursing policy. Our purpose in doing this is to help you think more critically and sensitively about your future in terms of the developing and unending practice of, and engagement with, the complexities of skilled interpersonal practice.

Your initial thought might be that the title of this chapter is a little strange; that 'CIPS in nursing' is surely all about technique! In some respects, this is of course true. However, the conscientious practice of CIPS in nursing which begins for you as a self-conscious endeavour should hopefully, over time, move you to a point where such practice becomes internalised as an increasingly refined automatic skills set. Equipped with this, you will hopefully and ideally do the appropriate interpersonal thing at the appropriate time, without thinking too much about it. Moreover, as you know by now, the skilled practice of CIPS does not take place in a contextual vacuum, so it is important to understand that this skills set will link to, and be informed by, multiple knowledge sources.

This chapter will help you, therefore, to move forward in this journey and to the chapters that follow in relation to a number of interlinked contexts. Within these, you will be able to situate CIPS in nursing in broader professional developmental, cultural, social-organisational, political and moral concerns. Specifically, you will be invited to consider:

- The context of CIPS in professional development at the level of *professional artistry* (Polanyi, 2009; Schön, 1987).
- How such professional artistry can be further understood at *critically reflexive* levels of increased organisational and political awareness (Grant and Radcliffe, 2015).
- How all of this links to the culture of contemporary nursing practice in terms of the ways in which the professional artistry paradigm (world-view) is in tension with the paradigm of *technical rationality* (Grant and Radcliffe, 2015; Schön, 1987), and the political implications for nursing practice that emerge from this tension.
- How this developing complexity of CIPS in nursing practice has further implications for the social organisation of healthcare practice, in terms of how nurses relate to each other, to other healthcare staff, and to patients, clients, service users and carers within their practice organisations.
- How exclusively technical rational approaches to CIPS in nursing practice may arguably undermine, trivialise and debase their worth.
- Finally, how many healthcare organisational members may be blind to this, underscoring the importance of critical reflexivity (Grant and Radcliffe, 2015; Morgan, 2006; Alvesson and Spicer, 2012).

Towards professional artistry in CIPS

The shift from self-conscious practice to skilled reflexive practice is an important transition journey for nurses. In terms of professional development, this represents the move from what Schön (1987) described as 'technical rational' to 'professional artistry' forms of practice. All nurses who persevere in the lifelong endeavour to improve on their understanding and practice of CIPS will draw professional artistry from embodied reservoirs of what Polanyi (2009) called *tacit knowledge*. This term refers to knowledge resources held by skilled nurses that are not easily made explicit or codified in language. Nurses draw on these resources flexibly in myriad different contexts, and act on them in automatic rather than deliberate and thought-through ways.

Theory summary: Professional artistry

Schön (1987) argued that those who practise, or advocate practice, at the level of technical rationality see the world in terms of *well-formed instrumental problems* requiring *specific technique* solutions. However, as most seasoned nursing professionals know, this model of the world of practice can be criticised for being simplistic and one-dimensional. Most nursing clinical scenarios requiring skilled CIPS practice are messy and complex, so attempts to reduce them to the level of straightforward 'one problem, one right solution' are doomed to fail. This is because nurses doing this are

(Continued)

(Continued)

functioning as technicians operating in a mechanistic way rather than as professionals engaging with complexity and nuance.

Polanyi (2009) described the remarkable, embodied virtuosity with which we often recognise and do the right thing in an immediate way, without being too aware of our reasoning processes that lead up to this, or engaging in a laboured comparison of the action we choose to take with alternatives. So, one consequence of becoming skilful in the area of CIPS in nursing is to learn to exercise appropriate action directly, in the absence of intermediate reasoning.

As an aspirational goal, professional artistry has long been recognised as crucial in advancing interpersonal work in the helping professions, through helping practitioners develop along a continuum from novice to expert practice. For example, this was promoted in all nursing by Benner (1982, 2000) and specifically in specialist mental health and mental health nurse psychotherapeutic practice by Grant (2010a).

Professional artistry and critical reflexivity

By this stage in the book, you should be familiar with the argument for the importance of reflective practice in professional nursing. Grant and Radcliffe (2015) argued that professional artistry, which in Schön's (1987) terms is developed through the process of *reflection-in-action* (or how our thinking helps us reshape what we are doing *while we are doing it*), should also involve the exercise of critical reflexivity. The practice of critical reflexivity takes us beyond personal introspection to demand that we are forever mindful

Activity 8.1   Research and reflection

Read:

Grant, A and Radcliffe, M (2015) Resisting technical rationality in mental health nurse higher education: a duoethnography. *The Qualitative Report (TQR)* 20(6), Article 6: 815–825.

Goodman, B (2014) Risk, rationality and learning for compassionate care: the link between management practices and the 'lifeworld' of nursing. *Nurse Education Today*, September, 34(9): 1265–1268.

In a small group, discuss the implications emerging from these two articles for CIPS practice, in your own particular branch of nursing.

of, and engaged with, the social and political contexts in which our CIPS practice takes place. The sociologist Charles Wright Mills (1959) argued for just such an approach in his seminal text, *The Sociological Imagination.* It is arguable that this past entreaty has often gone unheeded in contemporary nursing research, education and practice.

Clearly, relationships – whether between nurses and other healthcare professionals, or between nurses and clients, patients, service users, survivors or carers – do not take place in an organisational vacuum. We have learned from earlier chapters that environmental and other structural forces shape the nature of relationships in many ways.

This is an important issue, and gives the lie to the kinds of 'quick-fix' interpersonal solutions that belong to a decontextualised, technical–rational view of nursing. At all levels, nursing is political (taking place within power relationships), historically contingent (taking place at particular points in time, with associated policy and public perception demands on how nursing is perceived and practised), and socially and environmentally contextual (taking place within specific configurations of relationships, events and work settings). This overall state of affairs will inevitably place demands on you to embrace critical reflexivity, in order to develop your professional artistry of CIPS within the messiness of the contradictions that constitute real-life nursing practice and contemporary healthcare cultures. In this regard, it is important to be mindful of the fact that fundamental to the moral and ethical dimensions of professional artistry is the need to be human rather than mechanical.

Activity 8.2   Critical thinking

Some contradictions within competing narratives of the meaning and function of compassionate nursing

With fellow students, discuss the following argument, presented from different perspectives. One perspective is that CIPS skills can be taught on the basis of a simple rote learning, or algorithmic, model to combat compassion deficits in healthcare. This is challenged by critical social science perspectives. The argument focuses on the question: is the technical–rational assumption of CIPS as a set of skills that can be taught in a context-neutral way sufficient to remedy major interpersonal problems between nurses and the people in their care?

Within the last decade, in response to the mid-Staffordshire and other scandals, some NHS Trusts have commissioned 'compassion teaching'. The assumption is that such teaching will play a significant part in reducing the likelihood of future

(Continued)

(Continued)

large-scale interpersonal assaults by nurses and other healthcare workers on the people they are supposed to be caring for. How realistic is it, however, to expect that compassion skills teaching will make a major contribution to sustained, large-scale and meaningful improvements in nursing practice while the organisational systemic factors that arguably give rise to them remain relatively unchanged?

From a critical perspective, an over-emphasis on nurses taking individual responsibility to develop compassion skills arguably does little to address the politico-economic, structural, cultural and systemic problems that contribute significantly to the emergence of patterns of wide-scale abuse (Goodman, 2014). In this regard, individualising interpersonal and other abuses at the levels of problem (abusive nurses constitute 'a few bad apples') and solution (if nurses are taught correctly, they are more likely to choose to practise correctly) seems simplistic and flawed.

The proposition is that these systemic problems shape nursing professional identity at levels of healthcare custom, practice and assumptions. This is forever likely to undermine the best efforts and intentions of human agency to produce large-scale and lasting change for the better in healthcare organisational practice. In neoliberal systemic conditions that privilege staff compliance with organisational efficiency around hospital target achievement, empathic human relating will be accorded relatively less respect, despite policy and educational rhetoric.

Building on the argument in Chapter 1 of the power of environments to shape experiences and behaviour, different healthcare work settings will clearly have varying impact on the type, extent and level of empathic human relating that is possible in each. If the

Case study

In September 2014, the magazine *Private Eye* (no. 1374, p32) reported that a care worker in a private sector nursing home had been ostracised at work for several weeks, after complaining to her managers about residents suffering because there were too few staff to care for them properly. She described how she had been taunted by chants of 'loose lips sink ships' and expressed that she felt she was being driven out of her job. However, she was positive about her intention to turn out for a demonstration to be held outside parliament in late September 2014, of carers, health workers and relatives of those who had suffered neglect and poor care, lobbying for urgent reform of the law to protect whistleblowers (see Compassion in Care website at the end of this chapter).

argument developing in this chapter is accepted, technical–rational principles cannot be intelligently regarded as sufficient in providing a blanket solution to CIPS problems in environments that are culturally and structurally antagonistic to even adequate levels of nursing care. Consider to what extent the following case study illustrates one such example of this from the private healthcare sector.

Being skilled is not the same as being kind

On the basis of universal understandings of kindness (Phillips and Taylor, 2009), technical–rational competence in CIPS does not necessarily and simply equate to being compassionate. It may be instructive to consider this assertion in relation to what some nurse scholars describe as an international picture of nursing higher education curricula biased strongly in favour of competency development (Grant and Radcliffe, 2015; Shields et al., 2012). If this picture is accepted then, ironically, it may follow that CIPS competencies serve to conceal the absence of kindness in many practice areas, whereas critically reflexive learning might result in exposing this absence.

Clearly healthcare environments need to support such learning if it is to result in a better standard of CIPS practice. In this regard, it has been argued that critically reflexive professionals may often be perceived as a threat to the smooth running of such organisations, given their tendency to challenge fundamental organisational procedural assumptions (Grant and Radcliffe, 2015). However, if the status quo of healthcare practice around CIPS is to be scrutinised and improved, so that the people in our care and the colleagues we work with are treated more compassionately and kindly, it seems axiomatic that we need the presence of outspoken, critically reflexive practitioners in our healthcare and related services.

This message is strongly endorsed by Crawford (2014, p1), who makes the incisive point that the advances in technology informing contemporary nursing work, which relate to the need for competency-driven educational practices,

> *serve principally as a means of treating more patients, and are mainly used to get the conveyor belt they travel on to go faster [with the] … metrics, targets and production-line methodologies that have come to dominate our way of thinking.*

In this context, international higher education practices understandably and necessarily follow such advances in the aim of producing nursing practitioners who are both competency-savvy and competency-skilled (Shields et al., 2012). However, enabling nursing to practise in such ways, although valued by healthcare organisations, may also contribute to undermining the development of professional artistry in CIPS. This is because 'blip culture' encounters (Toffler, 1980; Brown et al., 2006), limited to a few minutes or less, may be all that is possible or, indeed, regarded as important in many contemporary, competency-focused practice environments which operate according to technical–rational principles.

Activity 8.3   Team working

Discuss the following proposition with your peers.

Frequently, nurses may 'say the right things' to patients/clients/service users, their relatives and carers, or colleagues, only for their facial expressions to give the lie to, and contradict, their words. The net result of this is that such nurses may at best appear shallow, patronising and/or insensitive, and at worst downright disingenuous. This phenomenon does not just apply to a small minority of nurses, as human beings are generally motivated to engage in *impression management* (Goffman, 1959). This is likely to mean that in pressurised, competency- rather than relationally-led, work situations the motivation to be convincingly seen to 'perform' compassion may simultaneously and ironically undermine such performance. Thus, attempts to disseminate CIPS knowledge and practice in events such as 'compassionate awareness' sessions in order to humanise nursing, may constitute a contradiction in terms. From a skills training perspective, 'compassionate' nursing behaviour may remain brittle and palpably false, hidden behind a veneer of professionalism, CIPS models and algorithms, which are more coldly efficient rather than authentically humane and heartfelt (Baker, 2013).

Hint: There is no one right way to approach the above discussion exercise. It is simply intended to help you work through and consider some of its points in dialogue with others.

Critical theory: The practice of CIPS in nursing

The mechanical practice of CIPS in nursing links to technical–rational assumptions about its need to be taught in response to perceptions of insufficient levels of compassion in healthcare organisations. This reflects a trend which emerged in the 1970s and 1980s around a lack of trust in public services. According to the moral philosopher Onora O'Neill (2002), this lack of trust resulted in healthcare and other public service organisations aiming for public 'transparency' through micro-management while actually creating cultures of deception. In this regard, Seddon (2008) argued that contemporary target-driven public service work cultures are frequently focused more on the need for public impression management and risk avoidance than fulfilling their care and treatment functions in morally coherent ways. In other words, many public-sector organisational cultures may be more concerned about how their services, and the people within them, look than about what they do or how well they do it.

The critically reflexive nurse as organisational role model

The argument in this chapter so far places a demand on contemporary nurses to strive towards functioning as critically reflexive CIPS role models, to challenge technologically and competency-sanctioned bad practice, and related organisational norms around unsatisfactory interpersonal relationships. In short, nurses should role-model humanness and kindness. We need to practise what we preach.

However, there are many ways in which CIPS-challenged organisations will mirror the poor and unsatisfactory relationships between staff members that, when experienced by patients and their relatives, result in complaints and the exposure of abusive practices. Ironically and tragically underscoring the need for nurses to strive towards ever greater levels of critically reflexive sophistication, CIPS-challenged organisations will often not be recognised as such by many of their members, who will employ the kinds of organisational defence mechanisms described earlier in this book to protect themselves from such awareness (Morgan, 2006).

In this regard, Alvesson and Spicer (2012) argue that a feature of the kinds of bureaucratic organisations we work in is *functional stupidity*. This term refers to a cognitively and emotionally informed unwillingness or inability to employ reflexivity or frank discussion about assumptions and related practice embedded in organisations. Thus many nurses and their managers are likely instead to regard the behaviours and experiences listed below as 'perfectly reasonable business as usual'.

Characteristics of the CIPS-challenged organisation

CIPS-challenged organisations are characterised by some or all of the following (and this list is by no means comprehensive; try adding to it):

- Staff not really involved in decision making, despite organisational rhetoric suggesting the opposite.
- Managers expecting healthcare staff to attend CIPS-related and other seminars and training, but viewing their own attendance as irrelevant or unnecessary.
- Staff finding themselves in 'I–it' rather than 'I–thou' relationships (Buber, 1958) (see Chapter 1), by, for example, being told how they are feeling or what they should be doing rather than being invited into dialogue about this.
- Colleagues and managers violating the principle of turn taking in conversations at meetings, through constant interruptions, with multiple people talking at once, while demonstrating a failure to listen to the person who has the floor at any particular point in the meeting.
- Staff receiving blip culture e-mails that are both confusing through an over-use of unexplained acronyms and lacking in necessary context, which thus do not

contain (and indeed may obscure) the necessary vital information for them to reply appropriately and in an informed way.

- Staff feeling compromised as a result of vital information not being passed on (to the ultimate disadvantage of patients).
- Senior staff and colleagues not responding to e-mails, or responding long after the need for a response has passed, thus neutralising the issues and concerns expressed in the sender's original e-mail.
- Senior staff being perpetually unavailable for contact with junior staff, by maintaining a 'closed-door' style, or restricting contact through managing interpersonal contact solely by time slot appointment or bureaucratic diktat.
- Senior staff constantly trivialising the concerns of more junior staff verbally, or even ignoring their physical presence.
- Staff being expected to account for themselves in a hurried way, in blip culture encounters, within which considered and patient discussion of context is sacrificed to 'bullet point' dialogues and exchanges.
- Colleagues failing to display normal civil courtesies, for example in exchanging smiles or verbal acknowledgements when they pass each other in corridors, or doing so in curt, dismissive or cold ways.

Activity 8.4   Team working

Informally survey your peers and practice colleagues, to gauge the extent to which they identify or disagree with any of the bullet points listed immediately above. If they connect with any, ask them how this leaves them feeling. Conversely, if they disagree with any, ask them how they experience their organisation as different. In both cases, reflect upon the ways in which their responses might relate to how patients, clients or service users are regarded and treated in the healthcare organisations they work in.

Towards a CIPS-friendly organisation

What would a healthcare organisation that was CIPS-aware, sensitive and competent be like? Staff would be much more involved in decision making at all levels of the organisation. Managers would role-model good self-development practice in taking part in training events along with their staff. Dialogue rather than monologue would characterise interactions between staff, which would also be informed by etiquette around turn-taking in conversations. Acronym-light emails would provide the necessary and sufficient context for messages to be interpreted easily, and all staff would respond to emails promptly. All information would be carefully passed on to its final destination.

Contact with senior staff would be more welcoming, less bureaucratically mediated, and with much more 'open door', relaxed and un-hurried exchanges. Finally all staff would be display civility and courteousness to each other, with coherence between their verbal and non-verbal behaviours.

Chapter summary

In this chapter we began by contextualising CIPS for each nurse in a developing professional artistry underpinned by organisationally and politically aware critical reflexivity. The discussion moved on to how professional artistry may be threatened by technical rationality in contemporary nursing practice. This was shown to have implications for the relationships between and among nurses and other healthcare staff and between nurses and the people in their care. It was argued that exclusively technical–rational approaches to CIPS in nursing practice may undermine, trivialise and debase its worth. Finally, the importance of critical reflexivity was underscored in the assertion that many healthcare organisational members may be blind to their own failure to role-model good interpersonal behaviour.

Further reading

O'Neill, O (2002) *A Question of Trust: The BBC Reith Lectures 2002*. New York: Cambridge University Press.

Phillips, A and Taylor, B (2009) *On Kindness*. London: Penguin.

Schön, DA (1987) *Educating the Reflective Practitioner: Toward a new design for teaching and learning in the professions*. San Francisco, CA: Jossey-Bass.

Seddon, J (2008) *Systems Thinking in the Public Sector: The failure of the reform regime ... and a manifesto for a better way*. Axminster: Triarchy Press.

Concepts and arguments from all of these books are used in this chapter. Reading them will help you develop your understanding of the interrelated ideas and arguments they contain.

Useful websites

www.compassionincare.com

The website of Compassion in Care, a charitable movement dedicated to addressing the plight of *victims of silence*. It is interesting to consider the extent to which the existence and activities of this movement are possible because it occupies a critical place outside of public and private healthcare provision, and is thus relatively more free from the constraints of technical rationality and positive public impression management.

www.missouriwestern.edu/orgs/polanyi/Duke/Duke2.pdf

This is Polanyi's original lecture outlining his ideas on tacit knowledge. It is hosted on the website of the Polanyi Organization.

polanyisociety.org

You can use this website to delve into more detail about how Polanyi's ideas were formed and structured into an argument.

www.wbuk.org

Whistleblowers UK is a non-profit-making organisation that supports actual and potential whistleblowers from many practice areas, including healthcare.

Chapter 9 The macro structuring of communication and interpersonal skills

NMC Standards of Proficiency for Registered Nurses

This chapter will address the following platforms and proficiencies:

Platform 1: Being an accountable professional

At the point of registration the registered nurse will be able to:

1.7 Demonstrate an understanding of research methods, ethics and governance in order to critically analyse, safely use, share and apply research findings to promote and inform best nursing practice.

Platform 2: Promoting health and preventing ill health

At the point of registration the registered nurse will be able to:

2.7 Understand and explain the contribution of social influences, health literacy, individual circumstances, behaviours and lifestyle choices to mental, physical and behavioural health outcomes.

2.9 Use appropriate communication skills and strength based approaches to support and enable people to make informed choices about their care to manage health challenges in order to have satisfying and fulfilling lives within the limitations caused by reduced capability, ill health and disability.

Platform 7: Coordinating care

At the point of registration the registered nurse will be able to:

7.2 Understand health legislation and current health and social care policies, and the mechanisms involved in influencing policy development and change, differentiating where appropriate between the devolved legislatures of the United Kingdom.

Introduction

Chapter 8 invited you to step into a place we have called 'beyond technique'. This is because we wish to discuss issues that are based in critical socio-political knowledge which is inadequately captured in much of contemporary nursing policy, education, research and practice. The aim is to help you think more critically and sensitively about the developing and unending practice of, and engagement with, the complexities of skilled interpersonal practice.

As you know by now, the skilled practice of CIPS does not take place in a contextual vacuum. It is important to understand that this skill set will link to, and be informed by, multiple knowledge sources often expressed in 'discourses'.

This chapter will help you to move forward and links to the chapters that follow. Within these chapters, you will be able to situate CIPS in nursing in broader professional developmental, cultural, social-organisational, political and moral concerns.

We will introduce some knowledge and ideas from the critical social sciences which paradoxically illustrate the point being made: that is our shared understanding and our knowledge of the world exists within and are expressed through 'discourses'. It is probably safe to say that most nursing students will not have been introduced to the discourse of critical social science and so this is new knowledge that has the potential to create within oneself a new level of critical understanding of the world in which people experience health and illness. Discourses are macro structures of communication because they 'exist' above the level of one-to-one communication even if they are *expressed* at the micro person to person level. Just because you don't use a certain discourse doesn't mean it does not exist in other social settings.

Discourse

We begin our exploration of the macro structures of communication, by looking at the concept of 'discourse'.

Concept summary: Discourse

In common understanding a 'discourse' is an exchange, perhaps of ideas, between two people involving language as the medium of transmission.

Discourse as a critical concept is associated with Michel Foucault. For Foucault (1969) discourses are *institutionalised* patterns of speech and knowledge seen and felt in 'disciplinary' structures, for example in the medical clinic or in the prison (Foucault, 1963, 1975). Discourses connect knowledge to power. To oversimplify, the concept refers to the idea that a discourse shapes, or constructs what we know, what we can say, and also reflects differences in power between people. The 'BioMedical and Psychiatric Discourses' can shape what we know and accept about health, and as powerful discourses can exclude other 'ways of knowing' e.g. personal experience or alternative therapies.

Discourses are more than mere words. A discourse, Foucault (1969, p54) suggested, actually *brings into being that of which it speaks*:

> ... *discourses ... are not ... a mere intersection of things and words ... the task of analysing discourses is to show that they are not just 'groups of signs' ... but as practices that systematically* **form the objects of which they speak** *... discourses are composed of signs; but what they do is more than use signs to designate things. It is this more that renders them irreducible to language and to speech. It is this 'more' that we must reveal and describe.*

It is as if Foucault is saying that 'objects/things/phenomena' do not exist for us until a discourse brings them into existence. 'Object' does not refer here always and only to a physical material thing. Objects may be abstract concepts such as 'hypertension'. This is a word, it is a sign, pointing us to a facet of our reality referring to the pressure of a fluid in a blood vessel, but it is *more* than that. It is part of the discourse and practice of biomedicine that *creates* a reality for us. Without a medical discourse that gives us the word 'hypertension' describing the pressure of blood in a cardiovascular system, 'hypertension' for us would not exist. Objectively, we might still have high blood pressure, but we would not be able to know of it, measure it or describe what it means. 'Hypertension' and its existence, is so taken for granted by us now because we have been immersed in this biomedical discourse for over two centuries since William Harvey (1578–1657) described the circulation of blood in his book '*De motu cordis*'. Hypertension 'exists' only because we have that discourse at this time and in certain places, especially critical care units and acute hospitals. It might be fair to speculate that for Indigenous peoples in the Amazon, isolated from 'civilised' societies, and without biomedical discursive practice, that 'hypertension' *does not exist*. They may still have high blood pressure, but they will not have 'hypertension'. The two are very different. Subjectively, they may not even have high blood pressure as they cannot name it or talk about it.

Thus, the clearest examples *nurses* will hear in their daily work is the 'biomedical discourse' or the 'institutional psychiatric discourse' (see Grant, 2015; Smith and Grant, 2016), both of which use phrases unintelligible to most people. Student nurses actively attend to this new language in their attempts to create a new professional identity, substituting words like cardiac for heart, gastric for tummy and neurological for nerves. In the institutional psychiatric discourse, 'bi-polar' is substituted for the lay term 'manic-depressive', and 'schizophrenia' for 'mad'. We suggest that the language of medicine and psychiatry is used to develop professional identity and establish professional power. We also suggest the use of such language can impede communication by excluding the ordinary person from sharing an understanding of medical knowledge as *they just do not have the right words.*

Students may have an insight into this process as they have a time-limited window in which they have one foot in both camps of nurse/HCP and patient. In situations where biomedical language is being used to communicate with patients, and neither the patient nor student had any idea what it meant, students might be able to improve communication by politely pointing out where 'jargon' is being used before they are socialised into uncritically using it themselves.

The language of the 6Cs

To further see and feel how knowledge is connected to power, and to understand what is brought into existence by words, it is suggested by us that the introduction, implementation, discussion and use of the UK's Chief Nursing Officer's '6Cs' is a newer version of a much older nursing discourse that emphasises the moral (Traynor, 2014), and virtuous (Sellman, 1997) and perhaps self-sacrificial (Pask, 2005) character of nursing work.

The 6Cs are the value base for 'Leading Change, Adding Value', a framework for nursing, midwifery and care staff. The 6Cs are: Care; Compassion; Competence; Communication; Courage; and Commitment.

The 6Cs is a discourse with knowledge/power effects. It has been allied to something called 'values based recruitment' in an overt attempt to police those entrants who wish to enter into nursing. The 6Cs and values based recruitment has a language, key words, phrases *and action* which function in a disciplinary fashion in that they set a boundary within which individual nurses should work. Transgression of that boundary not only could lead to loss of registration but also of moral character and professional identity.

The 6Cs have this primary function of setting out the boundary of professional nursing practice. They then have a secondary function of policing and protecting professional identity in the face of multiple public criticisms in recent years. The point here is not necessarily whether this is a good or bad thing, rather it is to illustrate how a discourse attempts to shape not only behaviour but how nurses, and others, see and police themselves. Foucault referred to the concept of **'governmentality'** to refer to self-policing. We return to this idea in Chapter 10. Thus, the discursive practice of using the 6Cs has the surface appearance and function of ensuring 'high quality patient care based on compassionate practice' as an *espoused theory* but it also has a disciplinary reality aimed at the self-policing by nurses of their own and colleagues' behaviours as a *theory in action*. To what degree the 6Cs have an actual direct causal relationship with high quality care, rather than a theoretical and intended one, is not yet clearly established.

Foucault's point is that such other discourses as the biomedical and the psychiatric not only *describe* something but also set limits about what that something is, what can be known, who knows it, how that knowledge is created and even who has the right to discuss the phenomenon in question. Recent discussions (McCarthy-Jones, 2017) about the nature and origins of schizophrenia imply the power of psychiatric practice in imposing its own understanding over and above other critical explanations and further, that mental health nursing to a large degree has uncritically accepted in practice if not in theory, this dominant explanation. Such discourses, within schools, hospitals and the military, are expressions of disciplinary or *carceral* power.

Later in this chapter we discuss in more detail the implications of the biomedical and evidence-based practice discourses.

Critical theory

Building on this notion of discourse, we turn to a 'critical discourse' that seeks to move us beyond common sense, everyday, taken for granted assumptions about 'what is' in order to think and bring about 'what could be'. This is because we think many nurses do not have a critical discourse to challenge taken for granted discourses that frame their realities and those of the people they work with. We start by discussing political discourses before applying the same thinking to health.

Case study: Learning from history

After Hitler's rise to power in 1933, the Institute for Social Research in Frankfurt moved to the USA. This group of scholars, the 'Frankfurt School', wished to understand the success of capitalism despite the conditions of the working class. The continuing, exploited as they saw it, position of workers in the USA, and specifically why they were seemingly acquiescent in the face of the Great Depression in the 1930s, needed explanation.

(Continued)

(Continued)

This group of scholars wished to understand and clarify the role of *culture*, which includes discourse and mass communication, in human affairs. Why had workers, made unemployed in huge numbers almost overnight after the 1929 Wall Street Crash, not risen up and demanded fundamental changes in how the economy works? What 'discursive practices' were dominant, what 'stories' or narratives were being told by politicians, media, academics and corporate leaders that kept them relatively quiet? What stories did they tell themselves and their families? In 2017, many were asking the same question following the election of Donald Trump (Goodman and Grant, 2017). **Critical theory** attempts to answer these sorts of questions.

In the UK, the story of '*take back control*' from '*faceless bureaucrats in Brussels*' was told in order to win votes in the Brexit referendum. One story on the side of a bus promised money for the NHS following withdrawal from the European Union. This followed the financial crash of 2007–2008 when governments provided billions to bail out failed banks. Following that, populations were asked to take pay freezes and accept cuts in public spending to reduce government debt. The story told was that (a) Labour caused the financial crash; and (b) the UK budget was like a household budget so debt had to be paid off. In this context arguments about paying for health and social care became more acute. In 2016–2017 there were many stories about a health and social care crisis, and a year on in 2017 the Royal College of Nursing claimed nurses took a *de facto* pay cut of 14% since 2010.

A question critical theorists ask is: why do populations believe these stories?

Theodore Adorno and Max Horkheimer were key members of the Frankfurt School. An important aspect of their critical theoretical work was their analysis of society and of 'power'. Who has it, how it is used, what effects does it have? Foucault's notion of discursive practices is pertinent, as analysis of discourses can indicate what power relationships exist in language and in action. The '£350 million pounds for the NHS' was an example of wider anti-EU discursive practice.

Critical theory is not just about power, it investigates 'ways of thinking' e.g. rationality.

In their book *Dialectic of Enlightenment* Adorno and Horkheimer (1944) argued our modern, industrialised, and increasingly bureaucratised world was underpinned by 'rationalisation'. Their thesis is that, since the eighteenth century, one of the defining aspects of mental activity (and thus also of practical action) was 'instrumental rationality', that is the rational calculation of means/ends to achieve a certain goal. This might be fine when applied to a factory production process but it has consequences if applied to human relationships. Key ideas associated with rationality are efficiency, effectiveness and economy. If these become dominant ideas in all areas of human activities, there will be consequences for the way we relate to each other. We need to consider who benefits from making these dominant ideas acceptable across society.

Adorno and Horkheimer suggested that as societies 'modernised', this form of rationality became more useful and valuable underpinning all scientific and technological development.

For example, in a palliative care setting, whose ethos and philosophy is centred in humanistic nursing theory (Wu and Volker, 2012), people acting and thinking about such goals and techniques as pain relief and nutritional assessment rooted in rationality, might end up overlooking the consequences for human interaction. This could result in certain interactions experienced by patients characterised by staff 'busyness' and professional distance (Kennett and Payne, 2009). Rationality also enables us to talk about people in terms of 'symptoms' and 'symptom control' – thereby reducing people to a cluster of symptoms.

Research summary: Rationality and science in palliative care

Potter et al. (2003, p10) described five common symptoms in three palliative care settings:

> *Pain (64%); anorexia (34%); constipation (32%); weakness (32%); and dyspnoea (31%).*

The language of the abstract of this article is an exemplar of rationality underpinning a medical discourse:

> *Patients referred to hospice and community services had the highest symptom burden (mean number of symptoms per patient 7.21 and 7.13, respectively). This study suggests that different patient subgroups may have different needs in terms of symptoms, which will be relevant for the planning and rationalization of palliative care services.*
>
> (Potter et al., 2003, p10)

Of course we can see that symptom control using rational science is very useful to people at the end of their lives even if there are other consequences.

However, rationality applied to human experience has some negative consequences. It is not the case that certain discourses are always 'wrong', rather certain discourses are powerful and support the position of certain groups. Foucault, among others, has argued that doctors have achieved their status and power in society largely by using scientific rationality as their underpinning knowledge base.

Greenhalgh and Hurwitz (1999, p50) described the problem thus:

> *At its most arid, modern medicine lacks a metric for existential qualities such as the inner hurt, despair, hope, grief, and moral pain that frequently accompany, and often indeed constitute, the illnesses from which people suffer.*

In the scientific rational biomedical approach the focus is on physical symptoms. Emotion or 'affect' is a distraction. Effective doctor–patient communication is only relevant in that the patient needs to understand what is expected of them, so they can comply with instructions, such as adhering to a regimen, taking medication, and so on. 'Compliance' is a word sometimes used to describe the patient's role in this context, with 'concordance' the more recent term for this.

One student nurse's comment in 2017 indicates how a rational, efficient, instrumental approach to care has certain consequences:

> *I have also experienced instances where nursing staff stop seeing patients as individual people, and focus on task and their own timetable.*

Activity 9.1   Research and reflection

Read:

Hillman, A, Tadd, W, Calnan, S, Calnan, M, Bayer, A and Read, S (2013) Risk, governance and the experience of care. *Sociology of Health and Illness,* 35(6): 939–955; and

Goodman, B (2014) Risk, rationality and learning for compassionate care; the link between management practices and the 'lifeworld' of nursing. *Nurse Education Today,* 34(9): 1265–1268.

In a small group, discuss the implications emerging from these articles for CIPS practice, particularly your own branch of nursing. Think of the role of risk and rationality as applied to the goals of care.

Max Horkheimer considered a theory to be critical if it seeks to 'liberate human beings from the circumstances that enslave them' (Horkheimer, 1982, p244). He suggests that biomedical, psychiatric, scientific rationality could be an enslavement in addition to class, ethnic and patriarchal relationships.

To begin uncovering what the social and political circumstances and discursive practices are that enable and constrain nursing communication and interpersonal relationships, we could start with discussing an idea from one of the Frankfurt scholars: Herbert Marcuse's 'one-dimensional man' (Marcuse, 1964).

'One-dimensional' thinking

Political and social theory is not core knowledge in nursing. Sociology has had to defend itself within nursing curricula. 'Critical Social Theory' is not a discourse routinely introduced or discussed. Nor is 'Climate Change, Sustainability and Health'. This may illustrate the 'one-dimensional' nature of much of nurse education (Goodman, 2011). This privileges, and takes for granted, some forms of knowledge as inherently more valuable, practical and relevant ('normative') for student nurses.

No one argues that biomedical, pharmacological and life sciences are irrelevant. The overall tone (discourse) of the NMC's standards for education, for example, sets out what is 'proper knowledge' for nurses, emphasising the technical skills required for leadership, pharmacology and clinical skills within a largely biomedical discourse, for adult nurses, that is instrumental in nature. By insisting on this knowledge, the NMC is exercising a disciplinary power over the education of student nurses.

'One-dimensionality' is a mode of thought that conforms to existing action, behaviour and world-view. It lacks a *critical dimension* that seeks to explore alternatives and potentialities. One-dimensionality accepts current norms, values and structures without being able to envision any alternative. It is not able to discover liberating possibilities, or engage in transformative practices. One-dimensionality is a state of being, a description, an adjective of 'what is' in opposition to 'what could be'.

The current structure of care for older people is underpinned by discursive practices that position them as 'disengaged', 'a burden', 'unproductive' and 'costly' to the Treasury and Society; they are the 'demographic time bomb'. In UK policy terms, we seem to find it difficult envisioning or enacting an alternative care structure that would humanise and valorise age. Alternatives to consider include the Dutch Buurtzorg model for social care and the concept of 'Gerotranscendance' rather than 'Disengagement'.

*Multi*dimensional discourse posits possibilities that transcend the current situation. We might then be free to perceive possibilities in the world that do not yet exist, or what Charles Eisenstein (2013) calls 'The More Beautiful World our Hearts Know is Possible'. Student nurses, as critical thinkers, are encouraged to think differently about 'what *could* be'; this of course applies to health and social care services.

Nurses are often asked to be agents of change, to be leaders, to consider alternative futures but they do so often within taken for granted frames of reference. Simon Stevens (2017) in the 'Five Year Forward View' echoes Derek Wanless in a previous report 13 years earlier, in calling for 'Radical Public Health'. What that actually means for you will depend on the boundaries of your thought and the narratives you believe in. Are, for example, the campaigns such as 'Change4Life' (2017) rooted in current norms, values and structures which emphasise the neoliberal discourse of 'individual responsibility for health' and limited state intervention? You will not be able to answer that question unless you understand what an 'individualising neoliberal discourse' is. Neoliberalism as an idea will be addressed in Chapter 11.

Case study: Neoliberal Individualism in action

A 75-year-old man with a history of depression and suicidal ideation is newly diagnosed with type 2 diabetes. He is obese and lives alone. His children are no longer in contact and live 150 miles away. He receives a state pension but has no occupational pension. He is encouraged by healthcare professionals to lose weight, exercise and change his diet in order to control his blood sugar levels. Within the policies of 'Make Every Contact Count' and 'Change4Life', he is encouraged to make individual lifestyle changes.

The wider determinants of health that include his social, economic and political circumstances are not addressed or even discussed. The role of local authorities, national government or health policies are not raised. Barton and Grant's (2006) Health Map never features in discussions around care provision by the Clinical Commissioning Group. The focus is on his 'taking responsibility for health' with support from health professionals. The concept of 'empowerment' is implicitly applied to his circumstances while at the same time the main input is centred around blood glucose control, medications and dietary/exercise changes.

Marcuse argued that countervailing forces to one-dimensional thinking *do* exist but they have to struggle against the dominance of the prevailing forces of control expressed through certain discourses. Marcuse does not reject the idea that contradiction, conflict, revolt or alternative action exist, rather that capitalism is increasingly one-dimensional in its application of technical rationality (see Chapter 8) to social and economic life, and this makes it increasingly difficult for populations to adopt anything other than uncritical, one-dimensional, ways of thinking.

For Marcuse, the prospect of 'one-dimensionality' meant losing individuality, freedom and the ability to dissent or control one's destiny. People in one-dimensional *societies* cannot distinguish between:

1. One's existence and human essence. We do not often consider if what we know of our existence has any relationship to what our 'essence' could be.

2. Fact and potential: this includes the material world in which you live which includes the everyday and the mundane. The fact that schoolchildren can buy sweets and crisps on the way to school is just that: a fact.

3.   Appearance and reality: What is the underlying reality of the appearance of the 'freedom of choice' in regards to food and fashion? In our use of social media posts, what underlying messages are there? What criteria do we implicitly use (reality) to value each other and what do we explicitly communicate in text and tweet (appearance)?

Marcuse would have us examine the culture of the society, e.g. our mass media and our social media outputs, to challenge our notions of 'existence, fact and appearance' to then think about 'essence, potential and reality'.

In other words, look beyond the actual words being written or spoken and think about what is *not* being discussed and therefore what is *not* being thought about as alternative ways of living. What is 'appearance', and what is the 'reality'? Bottled water 'appears' to be a healthy convenient consumer product but the 'reality' includes plastic pollution in our oceans.

One key aspect of our culture is the discourse of 'consumerism', including ideas about what constitutes the good life, what being a successful young man or women means, and what we should aspire to. Our acceptance of, or non-critical stance towards, a consumerist discourse defends us against calls for radical changes on how we live. An uncritical acceptance of consumerism, which upholds our 'right' to buy bottled water, could underpin our resistance to certain public health messages around lifestyle or legislative changes for sustainable health. 'Sustainable Health' itself is a competing discourse to consumerism (Goodman and East, 2014) which directly challenges notions of consumerism and an unfettered right to buy 'because we're worth it'.

We become one-dimensional in our thinking if we are unable to consider that health may be constructed differently, and if we are unable to consider and talk about the ways in which different forms of consuming behaviour, social relationships, working patterns, markets and technologies have effects on patterns of health and wellbeing.

Key characteristics of consumerism (Marcuse) and implications for health

1.   Individuals are integrated into society, content with their lot and unable to perceive possibilities for a happier and freer life. Consumerism prevents thinking about the wider determinants of health and instead sells an individualistic, lifestyle solution to health, while at the same time creating dissatisfaction with our bodies.

2.   Society's progress and affluence is based on waste and destruction, fuelled by exploitation and repression. This affects the health and wellbeing of populations in negative ways.

(Continued)

(Continued)

3. Freedom and democracy are based on manipulation, thus making it very hard to come up with alternative political action to address the social, political and commercial determinants of health because facts are distorted or not shared. Lies also become 'facts'.

4. The opulence and affluence of technological capitalism dehumanises and alienates. There is slavery in its labour system (e.g. zero hours, gig economies), ideology and indoctrination in its culture (e.g. 'there is no money'), fetishism in its consumerism (e.g. 'shop till you drop'), danger and insanity in its military industrial complex (e.g. threat of nuclear war).

5. Commodification and consumption: When everything has a price, becomes a commodity to be bought and sold in the market, when our prime social function is centred on buying 'stuff', we become too disempowered and distracted by bright shiny things to challenge the roots of *dis*-ease.

Marcuse (1964) argued that what is needed is to engage in the 'great refusal' – action and thought to challenge the dominant and controlling modes of existence; to criticise and negate the taken for granted; to hold 'power' accountable; to withdraw from advertising, marketing, consuming; to develop intellectually and culturally non-repressive forms of social relationships, through active citizenship, political discourse, culture and art.

In the next section, we revisit the concept of discourse to illustrate the potential for multidimensional thinking and communicating.

Activity 9.2   Critical thinking

Marcuse discussed the 'what is' and the 'what could be' – the difference between fact and potential. To help us move from fact to potential, think about what we currently have as 'facts' then think, what 'could be'? Be utopian, idealistic and aspirational. To help:

Fact: There is a 'social gradient in health' (Marmot, 2010) in which people lower down the socio-economic scale experience worse health outcomes and mortality rates than those at the top end. *Potential*: The steepness of the social gradient could be flattened out so that people at the bottom end of the socio-economic scale experience similar life expectancy to those at the top.

Fact: The normal retirement age is going up and people are working a 'normal' working week of 40 hours. *Potential*: The normal (optional) retirement age is 50 and people work no more than 3 days per week.

Fact: For most children who need mental health support and help, the average wait is 32 weeks for an appointment (Lilley, 2017). *Potential:* For most children who need mental health support and help, the average wait is 1 day for an appointment.

Fact: In England, the prevalence of obesity among adults rose from 14.9% to 26.9% between 1993 and 2015 (PHE, 2017). *Potential:* In the UK the prevalence of obesity among adults is about 5% with no rate of increase.

Discourses and health inequalities

In this section we explore the relationship between discourses and how we talk about health inequalities and poverty. Sandra Carlisle (2001) provided a useful summary on why there are 'contested explanations' for health inequalities using the idea of competing discourses. Your own explanatory discourse for poverty and health inequalities might be part of a more powerful narrative that creates realities for people through word, policy and action.

Activity 9.3   Team working

Discuss the following with your peers *and* consider what evidence you have for your position.

Does poverty and ill health arise from the failings of individuals or from failings of society?

Health is determined largely by the choices we make – to smoke, to drink alcohol, to be sedentary, to eat high calorie, sugar dense foods. Those who have long-term conditions in later life often were unwilling to choose healthy lifestyles.

Hint: There is no one right way to approach the above discussion exercise. It is simply intended to help you work through and consider some of its points in dialogue with others.

To explain inequalities in health, Carlisle (2001) outlined the:

- Redistribution Discourse (RED)
- Social Integration Discourse (SID)
- Moral Underclass Discourse (MUD).

Each discourse:

1. identifies the *source* of the problem

2. provides an *explanation* for the problem

3. identifies a *causal* mechanism

4. provides a *solution*

5. identifies the *level for action.*

So, within the 'Moral Underclass Discourse' we talk about health inequality and illness:

1. It is to be found in the lower socio-economic groups themselves (the 'chavs and skivers').

2. It is explained by *their* behaviour and experiences (smoking, drinking, unemployment).

3. It is caused by *their* lack of resources (which they waste anyway on smoking and booze).

4. It is solved by education and lifestyle advice (e.g. Change4Life).

5. Which is aimed at the individual (not the society or community).

One of the other explanatory frameworks for ill health and health inequalities is that of the 'material deprivation' thesis, which underpins much of the 2010 Marmot Review *'Fair Society Healthy Lives'*. It sits within a 'Redistribution Discourse', which suggests the answer is redistribution of material resources. Alongside this is the 'Psychosocial Comparison Thesis', which underpins such work as Richard Wilkinson and Kate Pickett's (2009) *'The Spirit Level'*. This forms part of the 'Social Integrationist Discourse' in which reduction of social inequalities and better integration of marginalised groups is important.

Material deprivation focuses on a lack of resources to support healthy living while psychosocial comparison suggests one's position in the social hierarchy, and the level of inequality in society, create psychosocial stress harmful to health. They are not mutually exclusive and of course might work together for some individuals resulting in poorer health outcomes for them. Being poor in an unequal society is therefore harmful, resulting in gross inequalities in health.

The 'Moral Underclass Discourse' includes the 'cultural thesis' and suggests it is the culture of certain behaviours, attitudes, values and norms that are the root cause of ill health. This can lead to **'lifestyle drift'** (Hunter et al., 2009; Popay et al., 2010) solutions to public health issues.

The answer in this discourse is to ask/encourage/educate people to make better choices and improve lifestyle activities such as stopping smoking, reducing alcohol consumption, exercising more and eating better. Poor people are disproportionately ill because of their poor life decisions according to this discourse. The 'underclass' make poor moral decisions and therefore bring ill health upon themselves; they are the 'undeserving poor'. The material deprivation they experience is a result of their own poor life choices; their parents' life choices. Material deprivation that *results* from being ill, preventing them from working or making better life choices, i.e. they are the 'deserving poor'.

Concept summary: 'Lifestyle drift'

This is the tendency for policy initiatives to recognise the need to take action on the wider determinants of health, 'upstream approaches', but which as they get implemented, drift downstream to focus on individual lifestyle factors (Hunter et al., 2009). It recognises social, environmental and political causes for ill health (e.g. the 'obesogenic environment') but in practical reality focuses on changing individual lifestyles rather than socio-political action.

We suggest that in popular culture, as expressed in broadcast and print media, the 'moral underclass discourse' is the dominant discourse used to explain illness and health inequalities. Nurses who do not understand the other discourses may therefore adopt modes of speech and explanatory frameworks for health that are 'one-dimensional' as they cannot think about alternative explanations or solutions. This discourse sits easily alongside a biomedical or psychiatric discourse, because of its focus on the individual and individual behaviour, rather than society or politics.

A biomedical discourse

Biomedicine and its discourse has dominated contemporary understandings of health in nursing and formed the basis of the NHS and other Western healthcare systems. The biomedical model claims to be scientific, objective and reproducible while the actual delivery of healthcare may be somewhat different. Many doctors now incorporate other approaches, for example Narrative Medicine, Complementary and Alternative Medicine (CAMs) and a BioPsychoSocial approach.

The main tenets of biomedical discourse are:

- Health is the 'absence of disease' and 'functional fitness'.
- Health services are geared mainly towards treating sick and disabled people.
- A high value is put on the provision of specialist medical services, in mainly institutional settings, typically hospitals or clinics.

- Doctors and other qualified experts diagnose illness and disease and sanction and supervise the withdrawal of service users from productive labour.
- The main function of health services is remedial or curative – to get people back to productive labour.
- Disease and sickness are explained within a biological framework that emphasises the physical nature of disease (i.e. it is biologically reductionist).
- Biomedicine works from a pathogenic (origins of disease) focus, emphasising risk factors and establishing abnormality (and normality).
- Evidence-based practice: A high value is put on using scientific methods of research and on scientific knowledge. Qualitative evidence given by lay people or produced through academic research generally has a lower status as knowledge than quantitative evidence produced by the Randomised Controlled Trial (RCT).

(Source: Jones, 1994)

As an 'ideal type', biomedicine considers 'professional knowledge' to be expert, rational and scientific. Lay beliefs, by contrast, are perceived as ill-informed, non-rational, unscientific and superstitious, and are thus devalued. According to this theory, lay people have beliefs and doctors have knowledge. In the biomedical model, symptoms are prioritised to the extent that they conform to diagnostic models. The doctor's job is to diagnose relevant symptoms.

We can see Adorno's and Horkeimer's 'rationality' in biomedicine as the focus is on objectivity, measurement and the hypothetico-deductive method. The development of science and medical technology allows us to 'see' disease processes within the body, so that sites of pathology can be pinpointed with greater accuracy (Helman, 2001). Despite being of huge benefit to people, Helman argued that this approach *has also contributed to a narrowing of medical vision – to the reductionism, mind–body dualism and objectification of body so characteristic today of the disease perspective* (Helman, 2001, p65). In other words, we can be reduced to numbers and physiological processes, we may be 'formed by that of which biomedicine speaks', i.e. 'the schizophrenic, the diabetic, the appendix', without a psychosocial context.

Activity 9.4   Team working

In small groups, list both the advantages and disadvantages of a biomedical approach and discourse to healthcare.

Suggested answers are at the end of the chapter.

Evidence-based practice discourse

Nurses in the application of **evidence-based practice** as advocated by the Evidence-Based Movement (EBM), and those immersed in a biomedical or psychiatric approach, may use instrumental reason to achieve certain ends as well as making assumptions about what can be known (epistemology) and what is 'real' (**ontology**). This can be a political project in that the adoption of certain EBM paradigms in clinical practice and clinical research can exclude other forms of research and evidence, and if taken up by those who decide research funding it can again exclude. Remember Adorno and Horkheimer argued rationality is a characteristic of modern societies operating in the background of thought and action.

For many, clinical practice involves the identification of 'ends', the goals of nursing care plans, and then the calculation of the means to achieve those ends. For example, an 'end' might be adequate pain relief or wound healing or optimum nutritional intake or safe medications administration. The means to achieve those ends often have already been laid down by others, i.e. the 'evidence'. The result is that practical action follows a means/ends calculation. This is at least the theory of clinical thinking. In actuality, action may be undertaken as part of custom and practice, routine or ritual, or deriving from clinical experience or personal reflection.

However, underpinning the surface raft of routine practices and communication, lies an ocean of biomedical rationality, even if it is not brought to consciousness at the point of action. This is part of nursing's 'lifeworld'. Nurses communicating with each other and with patients operate within this lifeworld of shared and assumed and often unvocalised meaning. They will not often explicitly refer to the rationality of the bio-medical empirical scientific literature, or the rationality of managerial imperatives, that underpins their daily practice. However, it is still there, operating 'behind their backs' as a 'generative mechanism' (Bhaskar, 1975) guiding thought, talk and action.

It is also the case that nurses will draw upon other various and competing *epistemologies*, 'theories of knowledge', in their interactions with people and for themselves. Exemplars of/for these are the vast range of what is called complementary and alternative medicine (CAM). Practical clinical knowledge built up through years of clinical experience will also be used. Nurses may also draw upon narratives, stories, personal and ethical knowledge to decide the course of action. There is thus a diversity and divergence from EBM in actual practice.

Holmes et al. (2006, p394) outline just such a divergence in an article aimed at clarifying what they call the 'politics of evidence'. They argue that:

> The evidence-based movement (EBM) is part of a wider political regime of truth; that it relies on potentially dangerous hierarchies such as the Cochrane taxonomy; and that it ideologically refuses to critique the deeper terms of its own legitimacy.

Holmes et al. argue that EBM refuses to consider its own assumptions about how to undertake research and upon what *theory of knowledge*, for example empiricism, it can be based. To begin to understand why, note that EBM is rooted in the biomedical approach and uses the language of the biomedical empirical sciences. The Cochrane hierarchy of evidence places the RCT as the gold standard for research relegating other methods and evidence as irrelevant at best or mere storytelling, '*anecdata*', which does not qualify as evidence at all.

In this debate we can see Foucault's 'power/knowledge' operating. EBM has power because it defines what can be known. In ruling out certain forms of evidence, the EBM exercises a form of power over what counts as knowledge, what clinical practice should be, who gets listened to and what research gets funded and published.

The Cochrane taxonomy denigrates clinical expertise, and similarly, qualitative research based on participants' narratives is 'systematically' ranked lower in value as 'evidence' (Holmes et al., 2006, p394).

Therefore Holmes and his colleagues ask of the EBM, 'What or who decides what will count as evidence? And what are the epistemological and ontological underpinnings of such decisions?' (p394). They challenge EBM to understand and critique their own assumptions about what can be known, epistemology, and what exists or can be, ontology. The inference is that critical reflexivity is never or rarely done by EBM.

They end by arguing (p395):

> The purpose of our critique was to spark epistemological and political debate over the implicit paradigms that impose a dangerously narrow and rigid system of 'truth', and impose it universally … Instead, we argue that researchers ought to encourage diverse and pluralistic paradigms and to eschew the rhetoric of the 'average patient'.

Student nurses will be introduced to evidence-based practice and will work within organisations and with people who take certain stances on what can be known, how one gets that knowledge, and what the proper form and methods of research should be. The paradigmatic and epistemological arguments may not be fully grasped at undergraduate

Activity 9.5   Research and team working

Read:

Grant, A, Zeeman, L and Aranda, K (2015) Queering the relationship between evidence-based mental health and psychiatric diagnosis: some implications for international mental health nurse curricular development. *Nurse Education Today*, e18–e20.

Goodman, B and Grant, A (2017) The case of the Trump regime: the need for resistance in international nurse education. *Nurse Education Today*, 52: 53–56.

In small groups, discuss the connection between these two papers and the implications emerging from this connection for CIPS in nursing.

level and this is not the place to discuss them at length. Consider however that this operates with a power framework because someone gets to decide what should be researched, how it should be researched, what gets published and funded.

Queering health

'Queer' approaches to healthcare form a set of loosely connected discourses, connected in one aim: this is to trouble and subvert those dominant discourses that are usually regarded as normative (Grant et al., 2015b; Zeeman et al., 2014a). The word *normative* refers to that which is unquestioningly accepted as 'normal' or 'just so'. Normative ways of looking at the world, critiqued in Queer writing, include regarding one term in a set of paired terms as dominant and superior, with the other term regarded as subordinate and/or inferior. So, for example, the term in bold in the following paired terms is often implicitly and explicitly assumed to be the normatively superior one in many, even developed, cultures:

men–women; **straight**–gay; **sane**–mad; **slim**–fat; **Christian**–Muslim

What do you notice about this list of paired terms? In the first place, they are 'either–or' and they are unaccepting of difference. Either people are culturally desirable (normal) or they're not, and difference isn't an option. Secondly, what is regarded as normal is never independent of local cultural value judgements and economic and political power.

Case Study: Adoption and difference

Nurse Sharon is taken aback on the children's ward when Darren and his partner George come to visit their adopted child on the ward. Sharon knows the NMC code of conduct inside out and has attended equality and diversity sessions. Yet her long-held moral intuitions based in 'Tradition and Sanctity' make her feel uncomfortable. Sharon voices her feelings in the staff room: '*I think that the responses from children who have experienced being brought up in a gay household have been negative; the only positive responses have come from adults. I think this says it all. It's the children that matter, not the parents. People just seem to be using this as another gay rights issue. Sorry, but what cannot happen naturally, should not be allowed to happen at all. It's unfair on the child. No matter how loving and caring the parents may be, that child will have to face people outside the home.*'

Dominant normative discourses tend to privilege groups, assumptions and behaviour considered culturally acceptable and desirable, while punishing that which is regarded as culturally deviant and undesirable. This has many implications for healthcare and healthcare communication and interpersonal relationships. One implication is the need for nurses to recognise how healthcare needs are intimately tied to oppressive, discriminatory, social, cultural, economic and political practices.

Case study: The murder of a trans women

www.mirror.co.uk/news/world-news/dandara-dos-santos-dead-brazil-9980288?service=responsive

(Communication with members of the trans communities was discussed in Chapter 7.)

On 15 February 2017, Dandara dos Santos, 42, was dragged from her Brazilian home, beaten up, and dumped in a wheelbarrow before being taken to a back alley and shot dead amid cheers and laughter. She was the fifth person to be murdered in February in a trend targeting members of the trans communities, in a global picture of 2,016 reported killings of trans and gender diverse people in 65 countries worldwide between 2008 and 2015.

Chapter summary

We began by outlining the concept of discourse and its meaning as discussed by Foucault. Crucially we understand that discourse is much more than an interchange of words and phrases. A discourse brings into existence those things about which it speaks. Discourses are not neutral, they often have a relationship to power and the social relationships that they form and are formed of. We then referred to critical theory and its attempts to understand culture and society, including language use and common expressions in consumer culture, going beyond a surface reality, or the 'taken for granted' assumptions. Again power relationships inform the analysis. Marcuse's idea of 'one-dimensionality' is used to illustrate how current forms of thinking and speaking can be used to justify and uphold the status quo whereas multiple voices attempt to create different realities. These theories underpin the illustrative discourses of biomedicine, evidence-based medicine, and discourses on health inequalities including the victim blaming 'moral underclass discourse'. Finally we outlined queering health in an attempt to identify binary pairs of words and the concept of 'normativity' to explore communication between health professionals and the people they work with.

Activities: brief outline answer

Activity 9.4: Team working (p178)

Biomedicine has advantages as well as disadvantages for the 'consumer'. For example:

- Biomedicine provides diagnostic categories and ways of dealing with pathologies that may help in the treatment or prevention of life-threatening illnesses.
- Biomedicine provides an easily identifiable structure which users can navigate to get their health needs addressed.
- Biomedicine provides effective treatment for many serious illnesses – for example, bypass surgery for heart conditions – which in the past may have resulted in death or long-term disability.
- Biomedicine produces experts who are highly specialised.

However:

- Some medical interventions can have serious side-effects.
- The user's view of why they are ill is not prioritised by biomedical practitioners.
- The use of technology may yield a diagnosis of disease which does not tally with how the user feels.
- Specialisation may imply a narrow focus and might lead to the practitioner neglecting interactional processes.

(Source: Open University course 'Issues in Complementary and Alternative Medicine')

Further reading

Browne, C (2017) *Critical Social Theory.* London: Sage.

Provides good background to this chapter.

Zeeman, L, Aranda, K and Grant, A (2014) *Queering Health: Critical challenges to normative health and healthcare.* Ross-on-Wye: PCCS Books.

A useful discussion of this topic.

Useful websites

For an outline of various approaches to healthcare delivery and illustrations of the variety of discourses around health, see the Open University resource 'Issues in Complementary and Alternative Medicine' K221: **www.open.edu/openlearncreate/mod/page/view.php?id=41623**

Chapter 10 The micro structuring of communication and interpersonal skills

Chapter aims

After reading this chapter, you should be able to:

- understand the concepts of Subjectivity, Self, Agency and Structure;
- describe what is meant by Modes of Reflexivity;
- understand the significance of 'Subject Positions';
- outline what is meant by post-structuralism, and governmentality.

Introduction

The last chapter on the *macro* structuring of communication acted as a bridge between 'beyond technique' and this chapter on the 'micro'; the intrapersonal (self) and interpersonal (with others) context of communication. We introduced some knowledge and ideas from the critical social sciences to argue that our shared understanding and our knowledge of the world exists within and are expressed through 'discourses'. Moreover, the skilled practice of CIPS does not take place in a contextual vacuum. There are liberating and constraining modes of thinking and power.

By the 'micro structuring' of communication we mean understanding the one to one, small group and our *own thinking*; 'talking to oneself', one's 'inner conversations'.

This chapter will help you, therefore, to move forward in relation to what we call the micro structuring of interpersonal skills and communication in a number of contexts. Within these, you will be able to see CIPS in nursing in broader professional developmental, cultural, social-organisational, political and moral concerns.

This chapter is heavily influenced by some social theory, a basic grasp of which is essential in moving beyond overly simplistic models of communication. It complements other perspectives such as Psychodynamic Theory expressed in **Transactional Analysis** (Stewart and Joines, 2012).

Specifically, you will be invited to consider:

'Subjectivity', how **Self** is created by and creates society and culture and how this then shapes what and how we communicate *with ourselves* and with each other.

Agency and structure, how our freedom to act operates within structures.

Modes of reflexivity, in which the self is talking to the self, using inner conversations, to decide on what course of action should be undertaken.

Subject positions, the way language and discourses position the self in relation to others especially when there are imbalances of power, and finally …

Poststructuralist and **Governmentality**, arguments that link language, knowledge and power to 'self-policing' of thought and action.

Core concepts to understand communication

The task we ask you to undertake is a rigorous and challenging level of personal, relational, cultural, theoretical and political reflexivity. We also ask you to understand some social theory, to develop a 'sociological imagination' (Wright Mills, 1959).

This is required to explore and interrogate sociocultural forces and discursive practices that shape our emerging subjectivities. It is about social and cultural critique, to address taken for granted and surface explanations for our thoughts and actions towards one another.

Social, institutional and organisational practices require robust scrutiny and critique especially if they are taken for granted as 'business as usual'.

Subjectivity and self

'Subjectivity' has a range of meanings but refers to our personhood, self, consciousness, perceptions and agency and how they relate to notions of truth and reality.

Subjectivism takes the position that there may not be clear boundaries between the external objective world and that of the subjective self. It is arguable whether the external social world, i.e. social structures, has a separate existence/being (ontology) from the self that is trying to understand it. Moreover 'existence/being' somehow resides in language and language forms.

However, **critical realism** (Bhaskar, 1975) pulls back from this position to argue that we are able to speak and understand 'existence/being' as having a reality separate from our experiences, thoughts, knowledge and language.

We argue that both perspectives can provide a better understanding of communication between people. We wish to avoid 'structural determinism' in which the nurse as 'subject, self, agent' appears as powerless and passive in the face of social structures. We also wish to avoid seeing the nurse as subject, self, agent appearing as completely self-created and independently self-directing. This is the 'liberal human self' critiqued in Chapter 11. We wish to avoid dissolving the human self into nothing more than language.

Social self

What we say, when we say it and how we interrelate with each other is a result of an ongoing process in which we are always interpreting the external world either quickly using 'mental short cuts' and emotions, or slowly using deliberative, analytical rational thinking. Daniel Kahneman (2011) calls this 'System 1 and System 2 thinking'. However, the 'I' doing this work may not be an objective, separate 'I'. It may well be part of a larger 'we' even if it feels like a solitary 'I'.

To take an everyday example, the 'I' that decided to get dressed this morning did so but with decisions that are exactly the same as many others in society. The 'I' was part of a larger 'we'. It felt like an autonomous decision, but one look around at what others have done will demonstrate it was a 'we' decision. What *feels* like an autonomous objective self, deciding to wear, say, denim jeans, is actually part of a larger *social self*. This social self is made up of people making exactly the same decisions. This is true for everyday and mundane decisions, and it might hold true for other larger decisions such as the way you are going to vote, or your interprofessional interactions or clinical decision making. We can think that we make independent objective decisions as free agents. But often we are part of wider decision making that has already occurred by others within social structures. Social structures provide 'conditions of possibility and constraints' for the actions of agents.

An example from mental health in the 1960s (Goffman, 1961) and nurse training experiences in the 1980s was the institutional care given to people who had learning difficulties or mental health issues. The language used to describe such care, the people themselves and practices carried out, were learned by new staff, and as they learn this language and followed culture and practice, they perpetuated the system. They created a new self as 'nurse' looking after people in conditions which we now might consider 'suboptimal' at best.

In this case the structure of institutional care predated the nursing actions within it that students learned. However, action taken by nurses can transform that structure resulting in 'structural elaboration', i.e. change. Of course lack of nurses' actions and speech *may not* change the structure and what we need to consider in the latter case is why it does not. Students' new selves as qualified nurses could be 'conforming nurses', perpetuating the structure, or 'challenging nurses' who change it. So, why conform and why challenge? Which self acts?

The role of our 'internal conversations' in this change process is vital. We must understand that the social world of nursing consists of structures, our agency and the cultures in which we work. Crucially, the role of what we say to ourselves, i.e. reflexivity, must be understood. We return to this later in this chapter.

Activity 10.1   Research and teamworking

Read:

Aston, M, Price, S, Kirk, S and Penney, T (2011) More than meets the eye. Feminist poststructuralism as a lens towards understanding obesity. *Journal of Advanced Nursing,* 68: 1187–1194.

Aston et al. argue that the meaning and experience of obesity arises from our social relationships. They seek to understand how *power* relationships work between individuals as they are constructed through social, institutional and political structures.

In a small group, discuss the implications emerging from this article for CIPS practice, in your particular branch of nursing.

More recent, high profile, examples of how cultures and structures impact on the actions of free agents include the Mid Staffordshire NHS Trust. The Grenfell Tower fire of 2017 indicates not just incompetence but cultural, political and social structural failures that facilitated, or made worse, the possibly negligent actions of people in positions of responsibility and accountability. We might ask: 'What were they thinking?'

Obesity and subjectivity

The issue of obesity illustrates the relationship between an 'external world' and an 'internal subjective self' *and* also that the individual's body is a place where socio-political meanings are applied. This is rooted in understanding that culture *flows through* self and vice versa. Being obese, fat, overweight, is experienced in a culture that has various meanings attached to those 'conditions' and the culture has various ways to describe a very human experience that can be internalised by the individual. This is sometimes internalised in a violent way, a violence towards self that is expressed in anxiety, depression, eating disorders and even suicide. The subjective 'I' that sees oneself as 'fat' exists in 'we' that has moral evaluations about being 'fat', sometimes backed up by the power to impose those moral evaluations via negative cultural expressions.

Lupton (2013) suggests a good deal of culture expresses obesity as: an *epidemic*; a public health *threat*; it is *dangerous* leading to the development of diseases such as type 2 diabetes; it indicates *moral weakness* and the *irresponsibility* of the individual for not taking care of themselves; it means *laziness*, not being the hero in a film; it is *unsexy* and *unattractive*. The politics of obesity involves shifting the responsibility towards the individual, known as a 'lifestyle drift' response (Hunter et al., 2009), rather than addressing the wider determinants of health (the 'causes of the causes') in the obesogenic environment.

Those cultural meanings will flow through the individual whose sense of self might be built on those meanings, leading to shame and self-loathing and paradoxically to comfort eating. Some reflexively resist this discourse, and instead talk of 'fatphobia'. They have a new language to challenge a dominant discourse, and thus their sense of self tries to create a *different*, less 'fattist' culture.

Thus, we are embedded within *dialogic*, socially shared, and linguistic practices in our daily preoccupations. 'Self' is *social and relational* rather than existing as a separate entity, i.e. as 'ontologically autonomous'. Two people discussing weight gain or weight loss do so within certain discourses, not all of which are immediately apparent. As soon as one person invokes the language of disease and illness then the other person can either accept or reject that frame of reference as they *reflexively deliberate* upon what has just been said.

The next section takes the idea of reflexivity to explore how our 'inner voices' can guide decision making and action in interpersonal relationships. Remember though, your self does not have a separate existence from culture and society, you *are* your society and society then arises out of you and others like you. Your *reflexive* self will hopefully uncover cultural assumptions and taken for granted practices.

Activity 10.2   Critical reflection

Identify something you 'take for granted', something 'obvious', something 'real, right or true'. Then consider why you think it is so. What assumptions are you making? What premises do you hold to be true? Is there another way of thinking about it?

For example: 'We put weight on when we eat too much' or 'drug addicts are responsible for their condition'. Then, 'nurses need to help individuals make better choices in relation to food and substance use'. Are you making an assumption that all weight gain can be explained by referring to the 'calories in-calories out' equation? Are you assuming that addiction is a physiological phenomenon related to the substance itself? Do you accept the premise that, ultimately, we are individually responsible for our health behaviours? Remind yourself that your 'fat and addiction' discourses underpin how you talk to people. Revisit the 'Moral Underclass Discourse' in Chapter 9.

Concept summary: Critical reflexivity

This is how we examine how one's own role, gender, class, profession, occupation, ethnicity, CIS status and socialisation affects the development of one's norms, values, beliefs and attitudes. How does all of that feed back into how one acts in society and culture? To be reflexive is to attend to one's own standpoints to critique them, to be aware of how they were constructed, to enable change and the potential reshaping of self. It understands how one's thinking can be *socially structured but not determined*, how it operates and how it may lead to courses of action. It is linking culture with self, seeing that culture flows through self and that self both constitutes *and is constituted by* culture.

Reflexivity leads to an examination of why one acted in the way one did. Or it may be that one has been so socialised into a practice that it never comes up for critical examination because the practice is so 'obvious', 'taken for granted'.

In the mental health domain, the 'obvious' and 'taken for granted' may be the background assumptions, values and epistemologies of biomedical psychiatry, or of cognitive behavioural therapy or the primacy of pharmaceutical approaches. The mental health

---

Scenario: Reflexivity

A group of students have been asked to undertake highly directed study in preparation for a seminar. The larger group is broken down into smaller teams of 4–5 students. A *reflexive* student nurse realises she has a common response in group work: to leave the leading of that group to others. *Critical* reflexivity on the part of the student reveals what the roots of that attitude and behaviour are. She might consider that her gender socialisation which valued and rewarded subservience, which labelled 'assertiveness' as unfeminine, was so strong that she internalised this view and has been acting out that patterned behaviour for years.

---

nurse who uncritically accepts practice may not be sufficiently critical of the outcomes of much of 'standard' mental health practice.

Mental health nurses and other state psychiatric workers are systematically stripped of their capacities to be kind through, among other things, being neoliberalised, classed, gendered, psydisciplined, and socialised to institutional psychiatric custom and practice.

(Grant, 2015)

Critical reflexivity requires examination of base assumptions, and how one's own experiences and culture shapes one's assumptions. Realising one's embeddedness in certain practice cultures and epistemologies may have both negative and positive cathartic effects.

Activity 10.3 Critical thinking

Mental health nurses and other state psychiatric workers are systematically stripped of their capacities to be kind through, among other things, being neoliberalised, classed, gendered, psydisciplined, and socialised to institutional psychiatric custom and practice.

(Grant, 2015)

What do the following words mean: 'neoliberalised', 'psydisciplined' and 'gendered'?

Note: neoliberalism will be discussed in Chapter 11.

Archer's 'Modes of reflexivity'

Margaret Archer argues:

> *Reflexivity mediates between the objective structural and cultural contexts confronting agents, who activate their properties as constraints and enablements as they pursue reflexively defined 'projects' based on their concerns.*

(Archer, 2013)

The way a student nurse *thinks* about a course of action in any given clinical context will be manifest in what they do, what aims they set themselves and based in how they see their abilities, options, *enablements and constraints*. They do so in an objective structural and cultural context. The clinic, the ward, the home is the objective setting.

Theory summary: Agency, structure, reflexivity

Agency: our ability to act independently of structures, such as class or gender, to make our own free choices.

Structure: factors such as class, gender, ethnicity, religion, family, occupation that could determine or limit an agent's 'free' decision making.

For Archer (2000), Foucault over-emphasised how language and 'discourse' impacts on agency and in creating a social world. Archer re-emphasises the role of the thinking human subject who has the ability to exercise their agency in objective social structures. She argues our reflexive deliberations 'guide' action (agency) in relation to the objective social world (structure) in which we find ourselves.

Archer (2003) describes four 'ideal types', or 'modes' of inner conversations, our 'lone inner dialogues' (reflexivity) that can direct action:

- Meta reflexivity (action follows understanding and values).
- Autonomous reflexivity (action is goal directed).
- Communicative reflexivity (action is socially directed).
- Fractured reflexivity (action is based on impulse, fear, emotion, habit).

Graham Scambler (2013a), in wishing to establish a theory of agency argues:

> *Humans ... are simultaneously the products of biological, psychological and social mechanisms while retaining their agency ... socially structured without being structurally determined.*

(p147)

Who, and what, we are arises socially, as well as from our physical biological selves, as well as from our psychological thinking and motivations. Society *structures* who we are without *determining* who we are. Family life structures us – giving language, culture, hopes and aspirations but does not *determine* these aspects of ourselves. There is room for *agency – the freedom to act as an agent*. A clinical setting structures us – giving us a language, a *discourse* (Foucault), acceptable modes of professional behaviours and explicit values (for example the 6Cs) in which we exercise our agency.

We might think that obese and overweight people choose 'freely' as agents to eat more than they need. Yet, they do so within the structure of the 'obesogenic environment'. We might think nurses choose 'freely' to inappropriately transfer vulnerable older adults, but they do so within the structures of certain management and interprofessional environments. So we need to see that agency – the freedom to act as an agent – works within a structural context, such as a clinical context, in which the social outcome is *structured* by that context, but *not determined* by it. This happens in the following way:

1. The clinical practice setting provides the external, objective, situation and context with which the nurse as 'free agent' is then confronted. The agent does not have a choice about this. The clinical setting provides situations of constraint and opportunities for the 'agent'. This objective situation operates in relation to:

2. Nurses who have their own internal, subjective, concerns in relation to their personal nursing theory and values, social realities (e.g. the doctor–nurse–management relationship), and cultural practices (e.g. managerial control practices).

3. The actions undertaken by structured free agents, in this case nurses, are produced by 'reflexive deliberations' (internal conversations) about the situation and their own concerns. Nurses determine their choices of practical action in relation to their objective circumstances.

The suggestion is that the mode of reflexivity adopted by nurses will then direct their communication with other people and a choice of action. Alternatively, 'not thinking', or not attending to one's inner conversation, could lead to the 'evil of banality' (Minnich, 2017).

Critical reflexivity and 'not thinking'

In Archer's typology, critical reflexivity relates to 'meta reflexivity' (MR); understanding who I am and why I think and behave as I do, then questioning the basis of that thinking. One considers, for example, the morality of action, the nature of personhood, empathetic consideration of the humanity of the other, the unity of experience with others and with the planet, gendered patterns of thinking, class-based patterns of thinking, or the possibility of heuristic thinking and our propensity to use emotion when reasoning. It means understanding perhaps 'ego states' and how we can be called into subservient 'subject positions' by powerful others. The meta reflexive, when considering what to do and before doing it, tends towards the perpetuation of 'rumination' considering alternative answers or different ways of looking at the question. One may think about, for example, professional and organisational patterns of thinking and how this shapes one's own thoughts and actions. It means challenging cliché, convention, insider jargon, technical terms and routine talk. It means overcoming the 'evil of banality' and accepting the 'life and death importance of thinking' (Minnich, 2017).

Meta reflexives are values driven over and above considering outcomes or consensus. Meta reflexives think about whether there is a correct course of action, what drives thinking before action, and whether their own thinking is free from bias, cognitive errors or delusion. Meta reflexives consider paradigms and epistemologies that underpin professional practice. They seek out an understanding of power structures and ethical positions.

In many clinical areas the pressure of work, managerial demands, time constraints, procedures and power structures militate against meta reflexivity. Socratic questioning would be an unaffordable luxury. The meta reflexive in this context could be seen as a nuisance, unrealistic, time wasting and inefficient. Meta reflexivity may also come at a personal cost, greater understanding leading to a realisation that one's personal agency is limited. Yet, without it we may end up doing 'what we've always done'.

In educational settings that focus on competency and skill acquisition, rooted in instrumental rationality and biomedicine, MR runs counter to the need for learning procedures, processes and facts. It also runs counter to the epistemology of much of evidence based practice, rooted as it is in often taken-for-granted empiricism (see Chapter 9). In clinical practice where the focus is on getting the work done, student meta reflexives run the risk of 'not fitting in'.

Elizabeth Minnich, after Hannah Arendt, in trying to understand the ordinariness, *the banality,* of the people who nonetheless commit or allow terrible acts, argues:

> *No great harm to many people could ever be perpetrated if distorted systems had to rely on moral monsters to do it, nor would any great good affecting many people happen if we had to depend on saints ...*

> (2017, p2)

while reflecting however that great harm *is* done (e.g. Mid Staffordshire NHS Trust, Winterbourne View): *people who are not thinking are capable of anything* (2017, p2).

When systems become characterised by suboptimal care, in which vulnerable people are subject to neglect or abuse, when inappropriate and ineffective treatment is nonetheless carried out, when people become stigmatised, marginalised and discounted ... when *extraordinary* events, sometimes known as 'sentinel events', e.g. lack of hydration, poor pain relief, pressure sore development, missed medications, malnutrition, verbal abuse, 'malignant social psychologies' (Kitwood, 1997) become *ordinary* events, it just takes a *practised conventionality, a clichéd conscience, emotional conformity or susceptibility to small scale bribery (or peer acceptance), a sense of isolation or a distrust of the reliability of others that works against taking a different public stand* (Minnich, 2017, p2).

Meta reflexivity, critical reflexivity, requires 'thinking close in' to get us beyond systems, excuses, and clichés to see the person right in front of us. Minnich argues that while the systems in which we work matter a great deal, the final moral responsibility for thought and action lies with the individual. We cannot assign all agency to economic, political and social systems but we do need to consider ourselves in context. Systems are *conditions of possibility*; they can provide structures for thought and action and help to create a subjectivity, but they are not causes of actions. We are structured but not determined. The task is to create a critically thinking *subjectivity* rather than a passive docile clichéd subjectivity.

Activity 10.4 Research

Read:

Goodman, B (2016) 'Lying to ourselves'. Rationality, critical reflexivity and the moral order as structured agency. *Nursing Philosophy*, 17(3): 211–221.

Nurses with high ethical standards sometimes fail to live up to them and may do so while deceiving themselves about such practices. Reasons for lapses are complex. However, multitudinous managerial demands arising within 'technical and instrumental rationality' may impact on honest decision making. This paper suggests that compliance processes, which operate within the social structural context of the technical and instrumental rationality manifest as 'managerialism', contribute to professional 'dishonesty' about lapses in care, sometimes through 'thoughtlessness'. Nurses need to understand these processes so they can critique the context in which they work and to move beyond either/or explanations of structure *or* agency for care failures, and professional dishonesty.

An '**autonomous reflexive**' (AR) does not stop to consider how their decisions will be thought of by others; they act because they think it is the correct course of action *for themselves*. They act decisively, trusting themselves sufficiently to commit to the conclusions they have come to. They are **outcomes** driven, over and above issues of value and consensus. They may fearlessly challenge power structures and ways of doing things, unafraid of personal consequences. However rather than engaging in meta reflexivity, they may engage in banal *thoughtlessness*, doing without this benchmark of critical self-analysis. They do not consider it useful to think about what other people think of them or their action. They could operate within their own interests and ethical standpoints that support them. They could end up 'lying to themselves' (Goodman, 2016), failing to think 'close in' (Minnich, 2017).

The student who is an AR may have developed a thick skin, and act according to whatever rules they see as right. If the transfer of a vulnerable patient is viewed as being in the nurses' own interests, for example if the following fits their goals: the work gets done, the team is appeased, management targets are achieved, it makes them feel good, then they will just get on with it. If the AR's interests are in line with patients' interests, their action will gladly disregard what others think. This might include acting with an ethical code that puts the vulnerable patient first, over and above the needs, wishes and requirements of the team, the management and the process. If they can think morally and ethically they could be a force for good. Their communication style could be directive and goal orientated and the nature of their interpersonal relationships are secondary to getting things done.

Communicative reflexives (CR) consider the needs, wishes and thoughts of others. They require validation by other people before acting. They rely on trusted others to complete and confirm their tentative decisions. They consider how any action will affect other people, and the opinions of other people become very important. They are consensus seekers and value this over and above outcomes or values. They refer and may defer to others' thinking and action and will not readily rock the boat. They are team players and value the smooth running of the team even if that team has lost sight of the purpose of action. Leading change will be through consensus building rather than personal affirmative action. At worse they may collude with a herd mentality as thoughtlessness, using conventional discourses that bypass the need for thinking.

The context of many clinical placements for student nurses values consensus and the consideration of others' needs. Mentors may look favourably upon a communicative reflexive if the boat is not being rocked. A communicative reflexive may be particularly open to professional socialisation and developing professional identity upon the consensus of 'what is'. A student working in a clinical environment in which suboptimal care occurs may feel unease, but if they have a dominant communicative reflexivity they may be very reticent to challenge and fall back on post hoc rationalisation for action; they may also fail to think 'close in'. Their communication and interpersonal relationships may be characterised as that of 'team players', as the 'caring nurse' because no one gets upset by any challenge.

There is one last mode: the fragmented reflexive. This person's thinking is so disoriented and unclear that thought and action are difficult or impossible. Thinking about action or the matter at hand brings them no nearer to an answer, which then intensifies the feeling of distress. Values, consensus or outcome thinking is secondary to personal survival in an uncertain world.

So, according to Archer, we have internal conversations. Our inner speech is rapid and often contracted into single words or phrases that contain a rich complexity of meaning.

Words and phrases have, 'semantic embedding in our biographies'. The word below, 'lifeworld', has a rich meaning to sociologists but means relatively little to others. The word 'compassion' has recently undergone a change in its richness of meaning as it newly embeds into the biographies of nurses. For student communicative reflexives: 'if we need to confirm our deliberations with other people, we need those to whom we express our thoughts to "get it", they need to share our "lifeworld", to "know where we are coming from". If they don't, then we have a personal trouble. If they do "get it", dialogue is smoother'.

Biographies are not individual, we live them out with others in a context. This context becomes a '*contextual resource*'. Biographies become 'intertwined' (student/mentor) in which the idiosyncrasy of shared meanings also become intertwined. This eases the sharing of inner conversations because we all share that idiosyncratic meaning. Hence we talk in short cuts, in jargon, cliché, conventions, half sentences. Archer calls this shared biographical context 'similars and familiars': 'they speak the same way, share the same meanings, draw upon a commonwealth of references and a common fund of relevant experiences'. Archer calls it 'contextual continuity'. It could provide the basis for Minnich's 'thoughtlessness'.

For a young nurse confronted with new decisions, such as her role and function in a new clinical placement, this contextual continuity is a resource. Engaging in CR, the students' internal conversation searches for many variations on important questions: 'What matters here? What should I be doing? How should I speak to patients or seniors?' If this inner conversation is shared with 'similars and familiars', there may be confirmation and completion of the inner voice's questions. If there is regular acceptance of the students' expression, this makes for a context in which communicative reflexivity can flourish.

However, if the context is 'discontinuous' from the students' own biography, there are no 'similars and familiars' who share the same lifeworld, and there may be serious consequences. For those who learn that their inner conversations make sense only to themselves, attempts at expressing inner conversations may then be rebuffed by incomprehension or misunderstanding. Efforts at making oneself clear may involve self-exposure; continued failure to communicate may well be hurtful and result in defensiveness. Students may resort to withdrawal or *thoughtlessness*.

The neophyte CR and AR nurse will have to navigate these difficult waters differently. It might be that the AR will resist the misunderstanding and the rebuffs and continue to answer her inner conversations in her own way albeit within the very real constraints of power, not the least of the mentor. Again we may hypothesise that a CR will try to fit in and learn what the 'similars and familiars' actually are, thus appeasing and pleasing mentors far more readily.

All this activity, communication and interpersonal relationships help in the creation of one's self, one's *social* identity, one's *professional* identity, as the self develops and grows and adapts to new situations. Cunningham and Kitson (2000a, 2000b) identified that self-awareness is one of five key domains for nursing leadership development, echoing Kouze and Posner (2011):

[S]elf-discovery and self-awareness are critical in developing the capacity to lead. And personal reflection and analysis of one's own leadership behavior are core components in that process ...

(p13)

Activity 10.5   Reflection

Identify a social situation and your own responses within it. For example, think about your role as a new member in a clinical team. Consider the degree to which you seek to understand what the consensus is and whether you feel comfortable in challenging it. How often do you catch yourself saying, 'Actually, I'm not sure that is correct ...' or 'I'm really not OK with that ...' or, 'I think this is the way forward, we should do this ...'. Consider the degree to which you feel comfortable if people disagree with you. Think about how often you take other people's feelings into consideration before choosing a course of action; do you always consult, ask, or involve them? Consider your role, your status or your socialisation in this. Are you able to say that you have a dominant mode of reflexivity?

Would others agree with you?

A note: these are ideal types of reflexivity and may be open to change within certain role sets and status. The status of Clinical Manager may be more fertile ground for an AR to flourish, if it allies with a role set that uses command and control directives. The status of student nurse may be fertile ground for the CR to flourish, especially if its role set includes the giving of 'compassionate care' and meeting the emotional and physical needs of others. In addition we may need to consider the role of *affect, how we feel,* when relating to other people. We need also to consider that we are social and relational beings with personal narratives and that this could impact on how our mode of reflexivity is manifest.

The next section explores how interpersonal relationships may be characterised by game playing and the taking up of certain positions to avoid, minimise or manage conflict. Affect, or feeling, might be an important motivation for taking up social positions and communicating in certain ways.

Professional interactions: subject positions theory

Refer back to Chapter 9 where Foucault's concept of discourse suggested that it can 'bring into being that of which it speaks'. The rest of this chapter draws from that idea.

Language can create a sense of self, who we think we are. We use different 'languages' (discourses) and therefore create different selves. We use language on others, to *position* them in relation to us.

According to Davies and Harre (1990) 'positioning' is:

> *the discursive process whereby selves are located in conversations as observably and subjectively coherent participants in jointly produced story lines. There can be interactive positioning in which what one person says positions another. And there can be reflexive positioning in which one positions oneself.*

(p48)

Note that selves are '*located in* conversations'. Just think about what that means. It suggests that the words, phrases, sentences you use to another person *puts them in place* to define who they are at that moment. Of course, the other person can accept that position or reject it and through language try to claim a different status.

Theory summary: Subject positions theory

Davies and Harre define a subject position thus:

> *A subject position incorporates both a conceptual repertoire and a location for persons within the structure of rights for those that use that repertoire. Once having taken up a particular position as one's own, a person inevitably sees the world from the vantage point of that position and in terms of the particular images, metaphors, storylines and concepts which are made relevant within the particular discursive practice in which they are positioned. At least a possibility of notional choice is inevitably involved because there are many and contradictory discursive practices that each person could engage in.*
> (Davies and Harre, 1990, p46)

We also use larger discursive *frames* which position who we think we are and what we think the proper course of action should be. The 6Cs is a recent frame outlining what nurses should be.

George Lakoff (2004) illustrated 'Framing' as part of political discourse. An example of that is 'Take Back Control', the 'War on Drugs/Terror' or 'Strong and Stable'. You can frame tax as either 'vital investment' or 'burden'. Nurses have been framed as 'Angels'. We can frame Public Health within a biomedical frame of reference (e.g. vaccinations), or a sanitation frame of reference (the provision of clean water and sewage services) or more recently a planetary frame of reference (Planetary Health).

At the one-to-one level, we build a sense of who we are, our 'selves'; we learn, use and adopt categories which include some and not others. These are often binary such as male/female, father/daughter. We then engage in 'discursive practices' that allocate meaning to those categories. The self is then positioned in relation to the stories that we use for those categories (for example as wife/not husband, or good wife/not bad wife). Davies and Harre argue we recognise ourselves as 'belonging' psychologically *and emotionally* to that position through adopting a commitment of a 'world-view' that fits with that membership category.

Think of the student/mentor positioning and the appropriate language used to ensure that you stay in one of those categories. Note how the language changes when teams go out to socialise and different *subject positions* are adopted. Consider the doctor/nurse relationship and language in the clinical setting, and then the same two people in a bar ... especially if the subject positions are now not medical colleague/nursing colleague but romantic advance/romantic response?

The concept of 'positioning' describes a fluid and dynamic sense of the multiple 'selves' or 'identities' one has, and also how these 'are called forth' and/or actively constructed, in conversations between people or in other discursive contexts.

Activity 10.6   Team working

Discuss the following statement with your peers:

> *Graduate nurses are too posh to wash or too clever to care ... I don't care how much you know, I just want to know you care.*

> (quoted in McSherry et al., 2012, p10)

What position is being actively constructed here? Where does the speaker want you to be? Does the role or status of the speaker change the subjective position you might take up after hearing it?

Hint: There's no one right way to approach the above discussion exercise. It is simply intended to help you work through and consider some of its points in dialogue with others.

Sundin-Huard (2001), in a discussion of 'subject positions theory', describes a case study in the UK in which the interaction between a nurse and a doctor over the care of a baby clarified the power dynamic, mutual expectations and discourses available to each of them. The case clearly demonstrated how the nurse was forced, in that instance, into a passive role by the discourse of the medical colleague. They had different views of what the baby needed, but the language used by the doctor enabled him to position himself as the more powerful, taking the subject position of 'scientific medical expert'. The nurse's language could not match it, and so she took up the subservient 'handmaiden' subject position. Thus the language used by medical staff can position nurses, and other people, into subordinate positions. One begins to think of oneself, at that moment, as less worthy/powerful than the other. Although now dated, this provided some evidence that suggested nurses had difficulties in making autonomous decisions and/or had problems with their relationships with medical staff.

Feminist post-structuralism

Case study: Male framing of cardiac symptoms

Think of a woman seeing a Paramedic, a GP, a Nurse Practitioner or a Triage Nurse in Accident and Emergency, complaining of vague symptoms of extreme fatigue and shortness of breath. Then think of a man complaining of pain in his chest and neck. History-taking involves asking questions and identifying 'red flag' symptoms, i.e. those that indicate serious conditions. A red flag for a serious heart condition is a man complaining of central chest pain radiating up his left arm and into his jaw and neck.

Women experience *coronary heart disease (CHD) differently than men. Presentations of cardiac pain for women can include vague signs and symptoms such as extreme fatigue, discomfort in the shoulder blades, and shortness of breath. Subsequently, the assessment, identification, treatment, and rehabilitation of women with CHD present challenging and unique opportunities for nurses because women* experience *a multiplicity of symptoms that are often not reported or recognised as cardiac in nature.*

O'Keefe-McCarthy, S (2008) Women's experiences of cardiac pain: a review of the literature. *Canadian Journal of Cardiovascular Nursing*, 18(3): 18–25.

Using the perspective of 'Feminist post-structuralism' (FPS), O'Keefe-McCarthy (2008) argues: *this approach examines the construction of meaning, power relationships, and the importance of language as it affects contemporary healthcare decisions.*

You might see the similarity in approach to 'subject positioning' and how language creates our 'selves' and our social worlds. The example of women presenting with vague symptoms however shows that it can affect clinical decisions, because we fail to spot the gendered nature of certain conditions such as cardiac disease. The reason symptoms are not easily recognised as cardiac in women is that the language of cardiac symptomology (e.g. central crushing chest pain) was based in *male* presentations and are thus descriptions of *male* experiences, but then applied to females. The *absence* of the language of (male) central crushing chest pain, and the replacement with (female) 'vague symptoms of fatigue', result in possible misdiagnosis. Language use and discourses can frame our decision making for females and cardiac pain, and it might also be true for people with mental health problems who are also from minority black and ethnic communities. This could explain the statistical over-representation of mental health problems of BME people.

Post-structuralism discusses how decisions are made through language use and the relationship between knowledge and power. It studies how we construct *meaning* in an encounter with each other, how the *power* relationship between the professional and the person can affect what meaning is constructed by us. *Feminist* post-structuralism adds the gender dimension to this by suggesting there are patriarchal discourses, patriarchal social institutions and power relationships that can marginalise and even oppress women and their perspectives. It asks questions such as:

- How does a (medical) language/discourse exemplify the relationship between power, knowledge and subjectivity?
- Why are some statements about health or illness accepted, and others are devalued or ignored?
- Are there androcentric (male-centred) biases in social, scientific, political and culturally established institutions such as the hospital or clinic?

Post-structuralism introduces the notion of power differences in interpersonal relationships. It is not the only theoretical perspective to do so. It is implied in psychodynamic approaches such as Transactional Analysis when discussing Adult–Parent–Child Ego States. You may have also come across Eric Berne's work 'Games People Play' using the 'I'm Ok, You're Ok' frame. What we would like to focus on now is the playing out of power games in interpersonal relationships using doctor–nurse communication as an example.

A daily experience for nurses is communicating with other professionals, especially doctors and psychiatrists. These interpersonal encounters are often highly gendered, that is to say nurses are still mostly female. An argument is that male ways of thinking, based on scientific rationality, cure, prediction, and diagnosis rooted in biomedical sciences is taught and learned by female as well as male doctors. It is further argued that medicine has been the more powerful profession and thus was able to 'set the agenda' in health and illness, and this agenda is experienced at the level of interpersonal communication between doctor, nurse and the person seeking help.

The literature on doctor–nurse communication and interpersonal relationships describes a complicated and ever changing pattern of professional working (Stein, 1967; Oakley,

2000; Goodman, 2012). This includes the idea that a significant source of stress for nurses is conflict with their medical colleagues. Not only does this suggest ways in which professionals negotiate their own practice in relation to each other *through their speech*, it also implies that there are impacts on the care that patients receive. Thus, it could be a factor in limiting or enhancing a patient's or nurse's autonomy (Goodman, 2003, 2004).

A few studies from 1992–2011 support the contention that interaction between nurses and doctors retain elements of game playing and the positioning of nurses into subordinate roles especially when it comes to decision making (Goodman, 2010). Holyoake (2011) argues that although Stein revisited his theory in 1990 and found that the game no longer existed, in contrast and in the face of denial by the nursing establishment, the game indeed does continue. Changes in the nursing profession have not been as far reaching as hoped by many in their attempts to professionalise it, thus game playing still arises (Tame, 2012).

If we can be positioned in a social order by other people's use of language and the discourses they use, and if our mode of reflexivity is communicative, i.e. we seek consensus rather than act autonomously, and if we accept other people's frame of reference as the correct one, or more powerful one, then we might adopt positions without realising it, or unconsciously police ourselves so that we conform to custom and practice. Our interpersonal relationships might become subservient, passive and acquiescent. Our communication might become non-challenging or non-assertive. The next section examines the idea of 'self-policing'.

Foucault and governmentality

The communication we engage in and the interpersonal relationships we develop are not necessarily immediately understandable at the surface level of speech. Superficially we think we know exactly what is being said and the effects this has on our relationships. The underlying theme we keep raising is how language is linked to knowledge and power, and that implies our interpersonal relationships are characterised by power being exercised through speech and action. This also applies to ourselves, that we apply power and govern ourselves as well as other people; Foucault called this 'governmentality'.

Governmentality is not to be confused with govern*ment*. The latter is a top–down hierarchical form of power. Foucault discusses how power is a form of social control, exercised through disciplinary institutions: the clinic, the prison, the school, the university, the hospital and the psychiatric unit. The production of knowledge and certain discourses may get internalised by individuals which leads to more *efficient* forms of social control, as this knowledge enables individuals to *govern themselves*.

Governmentality is the process by which power is exercised in a diffuse way so that we come to govern *ourselves and each other* without the need to refer to formal authority.

If a group can get their world-view, their paradigm, their ideology, their beliefs and values accepted by everybody else as self-evidently true and correct, then there is no need for external policing to ensure they are accepted. The recipient group will do that to themselves.

The paradigm becomes normal, in the background and taken for granted. It becomes a *normative governmentality* in which we can become so immersed that we become blind to it, as its worldview is just 'obvious'. It is 'normal'. In the previous chapter we saw how an evidence-based practice paradigm was critiqued for its uncritical stance to its own assumed normality. We suggest 'paradigms' such as the 6Cs could similarly be critiqued for their uncritical and assumed normality. Many potential recruits to nursing have so internalised the 6Cs they effectively are policing themselves in order to gain entry to the profession.

In healthcare delivery we have 'paradigms', that to their practitioners are just obvious:

- Biomedicine
- Institutional psychiatry
- Bio-psycho-social
- Person-centred care
- Complementary and alternative therapies (this group is diverse and has multiple ways of knowing).

We suggest that *normative governmentality* exists to a great degree in that biomedicine and institutional psychiatry are understood by many as 'just how things should be'.

Some will object and argue that biomedicine is outdated and no longer practised, and indeed many doctors are using other approaches, such as 'narrative medicine'. Whatever the actuality of the case, normative governmentality can blind us to what we are actually doing because we take it for granted, using cliché, jargon and convention.

Self-policing is not new. People experiencing delusion thoughts have to police themselves often with medications. The over-reliance of drugs can individualise health problems and seeks solutions in changing individual behaviour via medication use. In this manner we may disregard the wider determinants of health and focus our communication and interpersonal relationships at this micro level of medications management.

If we turn this gaze towards everyday nursing practices, we might ask questions about the fundamental nature of the nurse–person interaction in various clinical fields and wonder about the degree of self-policing we are asking for.

Roberts (2005) examines how power and knowledge are central to the process by which human beings are 'made subjects' and, therefore, how 'psychiatric identities' are produced. He argues that the power of psychiatric categorisations and diagnoses are such that they can come to utterly overwhelm a person's identity, citing R.D. Laing

(1990) who suggested that: *No one has schizophrenia, like having a cold. The patient has not got schizophrenia. He is schizophrenic* (p34).

Roberts goes on to suggest that:

> *A person is not thought to have schizophrenia while remaining 'essentially' the same; rather, schizophrenia is thought to 'split' or 'fragment' the very 'essence', the very being, of a person. To give a person a diagnosis of schizophrenia, therefore, is not to give a person one identity amongst others; instead, it is to suggest that a person is schizophrenic, that schizophrenia determines the very being of that person.*

The diagnosis becomes a 'master status', framing subjective experience, interpersonal relationships and communication. The nurse and the person they work with can easily accept that identity and reinforce it in their language and relationships; if they do so they are exercising 'governmentality', policing themselves to conform to others' expectations.

Chapter summary

We have introduced theory about subjectivity, self, structure, agency, reflexive deliberations, thoughtlessness, subject positions, post-structuralism and governmentality in an attempt to describe how the micro communications and interpersonal relationships we engage in, must not be understood as neutral encounters between equal partners, even if on the surface they appear so. We suggest that our selves are social, relational and perhaps multiple. In exercising our personal agency we help to create that which creates us – culture and society. Archer tries to examine why we chose a course of action based on an inner conversation that occurs in particular social settings that for us at that point are fixed. Yet in acting we may begin to change that social setting. However, if we fail to think about our context and our assumptions we may perpetuate systems that cause harm, and worse if that system is 'normal' we may deceive ourselves, police ourselves, and not challenge the taken for granted. In this manner communication becomes a mere transaction and our interpersonal relationships can be become dehumanised and myopic, seeing faults in individuals rather than arising also within social structures.

Further reading

The following publications provide some further explanation of the social theory that influenced this chapter.

Archer, M (2003) *Structure, Agency and the Internal Conversation.* Cambridge: Cambridge University Press.

Archer, M et al. (2016) What is critical realism? *Perspectives*, 38(2): 4–9.

Minnich, E (2017) *The Evil of Banality: On the life and death importance of thinking.* New York: Rowman and Littlefield.

Rabinow, P (1991) *The Foucault Reader: An introduction to Foucault's thought.* London: Penguin.

Useful websites

These provide some further explanation of the social theory that influenced this chapter.

Critical realism: **https://centreforcriticalrealism.com/about-critical-realism/basic-critical-realism/**

Foucault: **www.theory.org.uk/ctr-fouc.htm**

Subject positions: **www.massey.ac.nz/~alock/theory/subpos.htm**

Chapter 11 The political context of communication and interpersonal skills

Introduction

Cunningham and Kitson (2000a, 2000b) identified 'political awareness' as one of the five domains for leadership development for nurses. As such, it is necessary for all nurses to develop this awareness to reflect on how it affects communication and interpersonal relationships.

We will briefly introduce *some* of the 'politics of health' after a very brief outline of political ideologies and positions.

A very important thing to note is that politics is often about a 'narrative'; a *story* about how the world is and how it should be. These stories are communicated via myriad methods of interpersonal and mass media of communication. What you think about any given issue is rooted in deep seated and often unexamined stories you hold to be true. People consciously and unconsciously use these stories to justify health policy and to set the direction of health policy. For example, the question of whether patients who miss GP appointments should be charged is underpinned by deeper intuitions about fairness and moral responsibility.

We emphasise the point that what we are told, and what we say, about health and social care funding, about determinants of health, about what causes health inequalities and how people should change behaviour for health, is often done through stories rooted in taken for granted political positions, moral intuitions and 'frames'. Therefore it is crucial we begin to examine our own stories and assumptions if we wish to be active, informed participants in health policy at local, national or international level.

We begin by briefly addressing the basic question 'What is politics?' We will ask you to consider your own politics and to help with that we outline common 'isms' and the narratives that go with them. We discuss the idea of the 'liberal human self', and why that understanding might be important for our understanding of health behaviours and health inequalities. Obesity will be used as an example of competing discourses that underpin policy.

The relevance for communication and interpersonal skills is that:

- Nurses have the capacity to use the political element of their role to implement and amplify good policy as well as question/challenge the bad.
- Personal biases/deeply held political views can manifest within the nursing role, sometimes unconsciously.
- A nurse's job as a regulated profession occupies a significant position within society, and provides an authoritative voice. This means the public has deeply held views of 'the nurse'. This view/authority is inherently bound up in politics which are then manifest in nurses' professional messages.
- Clinical practice is guided by a large body of policy, e.g. from the *Code*, Make Every Contact Count, the 6Cs and the Health and Social Care Act 2012. Therefore it is important to understand some of the assumptions, their political positions and their implications.
- If you are unsure of what certain political 'isms' are, we suggest that you undertake the first activity to get an idea of what they might be. You do not have be an expert in political philosophies, but it does help if you begin to clarify in your mind the range of positions taken by people and policy makers.

Activity 11.1 Critical thinking

Understanding 'isms' For an excellent brief introduction and overview of liberalism, conservatism and socialism, access the podcast 'Liberalism's Horrible Year' at **www.bbc.co.uk/programmes/b085b73s** from Radio 4's 'The Briefing Room'.

Another brief resource can be found here: 'Quick Definitions of Political Ideologies: The –Isms'. **www.dummies.com/education/politics-government/ quick-definitions-of-political-ideologies-the-isms/**.

The book is *British Politics for Dummies* by Knight, J and Pattison, M (2015) Wiley, London.

As this an exercise individual to you, there is no answer at the end of the chapter.

What might 'politics' mean?

The Greek word 'polis' means city or community; 'politis' means citizen; 'Politiká' means 'affairs of the cities'.

Chafee et al. (2012) suggested that politics can be defined simply as:

the process of influencing the scarce allocation of resources.

(p5)

'Resource allocation' requires us to engage with critical analyses of power and the legitimacy of the exercise of power. This is because the exercise of power decides who gets what, how they get it, when they get it and how it is paid for. Later in the chapter, you will be asked to consider the story of a GP and her patient with MS. The story is about who has the power to decide what support the patient receives. It calls into question the legitimacy of the exercise of that power.

We are not restricting politics to Parliament. People are engaged in politics without ever joining parties or stepping foot inside the palace of Westminster. Discussions about resource allocation take place in an organisation's clinical area as well as the boardroom.

The exercise of power involves designing policies and structures for health and social care. The NHS itself is a very clear example of the translation of political views into actual policy through the exercise of power. How we continue to treat frail older people, children, those with learning disabilities and with acute mental health issues is thus political.

- We suggest that 'health is political'.
- We also suggest healthcare professional practice is political.

So a 'politics of health' is about:

1. The allocation of resources.
2. Understanding power and its exercise.
3. Development and implementation of health and social care policy.
4. Citizenship, activism, and professional practice beyond Parliament.

The next section is to help you identify your own, and others', political assumptions and values which impact on how you would allocate resources and design health policies.

The Political Compass

One very useful way to think about political positions is that of the 'Political Compass' which uses two continuums – the Economic and the Social: the words 'Left/Right' are about *Economic* position. The *Social* positions are 'Authoritarian/Liberal' or, as George Lakoff (2014) argues, the 'Strict Father/Nurturing Parent' narratives.

Theory summary: 'Austerity' as resource allocation

Since 2010, 'austerity' was about attempts at controlling UK Government spending to reduce the yearly deficit – the difference between what the Government receives and what it plans to spend in that one year. This aimed to address the *total national debt*, i.e. the sum total of all the yearly deficits added together. It has been aimed at public services, with the NHS to a degree being 'protected' from actual cuts.

Issues with austerity

The National Audit Office report (2018) states:

1. *The Department (of Health) cannot demonstrate that the sector is sustainably funded. Between 2010/11 and 2016/17, spending on care by Local Authorities reduced by 5.3% in real terms.*
2. *Four fifths of LAs are paying fees to providers that are below the benchmark costs of care.*

The *Financial Times* reported on 4 July 2017 that the Local Government Association called for an end to 'austerity' arguing that their core funding will be cut by 77% between 2015 and 2020 amid uncertainty about what will replace it.

See: **www.ft.com/content/9c6b5284-6000-11e7-91a7-502f7ee26895**

To connect the issue of LA funding with healthcare, see 'Is your Local Council going bust?' available at **www.bbc.co.uk/programmes/b09qb0l0**. This is part of the excellent series 'The Briefing Room' by the BBC's Radio 4. Listen to it as a podcast.

You might want to access the Government's response to these criticisms; particularly listen to Ministers' statements on the NHS and social care available across a wide range of media.

You need to bear this in mind when you hear words such as 'left wing' or 'authoritarian'. You will have a position somewhere in these quadrants based on your ideas about the role of the State on economics *and* the degree of individual freedom you value. If you have taken the test you will know where you are. Note that action for public health is often based in the positions taken by policy makers on these two continuums. We will return to this below when considering action on the social determinants of health.

Activity 11.2   Critical thinking

What is your political position? Find out here: **www.politicalcompass.org**. We really recommend that you do this.

The Political Compass: Economic and Social Politics

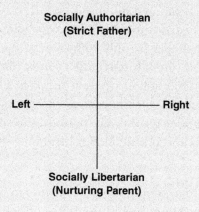

Conservatism and Socialism

Associated with the *Economic* continuum in common language are the two traditional or dominant 'isms': Conservatism – The 'Right', and Socialism – The 'Left'.

Although these 'isms' are linked to the Conservative and Labour parties respectively, it would be a mistake to think the parties are very discrete ideologically, completely separated by their views on (1) the State and the Economy and (2) Society and the Individual. A focus on this party binary also erases discussion about other UK parties such as the Liberal Democrats and the Green Party. For simplification, bearing in mind this is not a textbook on politics, we will focus on these binaries as 'ideal types' whereas reality is far more complicated.

An important rift is about the proper role of the State in people's lives, i.e. the *Social* continuum – you may hear this in the arguments over public health measures. The common phrase is 'nanny state interference' used by those who emphasise personal responsibility and liberty (Socially Libertarian). These rifts at times mean that there is as much of a difference *within* a party as there is between them, and that some MPs have more in common with their opposite party MPs than those in their own parties on certain issues.

The NHS has since 1948 been an agreed issue, but today rifts within and between parties about what it is and what it should be, and how it should be funded, e.g. more private insurance, are appearing.

Common ideological divides and the stories that go with them

1. **Small State (conservative, Right) v Big State (socialist, Left)** – to what degree should the State be involved in providing healthcare?

The first story (Right) is: 'Public spending should be cut right back, the State should not be in the business of running a monopoly health care service' (Libertarian Right). Some argue (Adam Smith Institute, 2017, see **www.adamsmith.org/policy**) that total spending by government should be only 10% of what the country produces (known as GDP) rather than the 40% the UK currently spends. This would mean reducing government spending from £700 billion per year down to £125 billion per year, reducing NHS spending by 75%. Ideally, the State *should not* provide health services and should only be the emergency funder for the very poor. In this scenario, individuals and charities and social enterprises and private health insurance should fill the funding gap left by the government.

The other (Left) story is that, 'There should continue to be State funding and provision paid for out of general taxation: free at the point of delivery, equitable, with universal and comprehensive healthcare' (i.e. an NHS). It is the proper role of the State to provide healthcare services (Left). You will hear this in discussions about the 'NHS Funding Crisis' which asks the government to increase levels of funding to the NHS.

This divide also is expressed as **Free Market (conservative, Right) v State Intervention (socialist, Left)**. One side says there should be a free market in health provision, including private health insurance and 'any willing provider' should be allowed to bid for health service contracts in competition with other providers. Health service provision should be delivered by private companies via a market mechanism. As against: State planning, funding and monopoly provision of health services.

Public health should either (a) have only a minimal educational role to prevent nannying interference in people's lives *or* (b) it should be a comprehensive, interventionist service involving education, community development, government funded projects and legislation.

2. **Tax is theft** (so lower tax) (**conservative, Libertarian Right**) **v tax is investment (socialist, Authoritarian Left)** (so reform or increase tax). The first story is that tax is coercion, is force, to pay for something that the individual may not want. Only the individual is able and is best placed to make those choices (Libertarian). As against: To provide clean water, sewerage and myriad other public health interventions to keep a population healthy, tax is a necessary investment (Authoritarian) otherwise we cannot provide care for older people, learning disabilities, child services or protect populations from epidemics.

3. **Individual Responsibility (conservative, Libertarian) v Collectivist Responsibility (socialist, Authoritarian)**. The first story is that, 'There is no such thing as society, only individuals and families'. Therefore each of us has to look after ourselves and

our immediate family. We must make provision for our own health, education, housing, social care and provide that care for our own children, ourselves and our own parents. We must adopt healthy lifestyles and take individual responsibility for health. As against: There *is* such a thing as society, and if there are people 'left behind' because of chance and social conditions, then we all suffer. So, to ensure everyone has a chance to enjoy a long healthy life and care in later life, there is a social responsibility to provide housing, education and health and social care services paid for out of general taxation. We should not go back to the situation in which the five giant evils of 'Want, Ignorance, Idleness, Disease and Squalor' prevailed and as outlined in the Beveridge Report of 1942.

4. **Socially Authoritarian (conservative) v Socially Liberal (socialist).** The first conservative story ('Strict Father') is that the family is properly a man and a woman bringing up children; it is heterosexual. The proper male role is to 'protect and provide'. There are essential male/female differences. Sexuality is binary, it is not fluid. Transgender issues are aberrations or arise as biological abnormalities. The Sanctity of Life takes precedence over Women's Choice; thus abortion should be illegal or very restricted. Marriage is a sacred sacrament. Feminism is a social threat beyond asking for equal opportunities in the workplace. There is no such thing as patriarchy. Women are natural carers, emotional and nurturers. Men are more rational and practical. Nursing suits women more, so it is no accident that it is a female dominated occupation. The moral intuitions of Tradition, Hierarchy and Authority (Haidt, 2012) in social life are especially important values, expressed for example in support for the monarchy. The socially liberal position ('Nurturing Parent') is almost the binary opposite on all counts.

The following divides are less directly relevant for healthcare policy and practice.

- **Patriotism,** Britain First – **Internationalist,** pro EU.
- **Immigration is a threat – Immigration is a bonus**
- **Brexit: Leave – Remain** is an issue that cuts across left/right conservative/socialist divides.

Activity 11.3 Reflection

Group work. Get together and take the political compass test and/or discuss the narratives above. Note where you agree and where you disagree. Try to think why you have staked out your positions. What deep seated values do you think you are invoking? Make a list. You might want to follow this up by reading up on Jonathan Haidt's 'Moral Foundations Theory' briefly mentioned later in the chapter. The website is listed at the end.

As this exercise is individual to you there is no answer at the end of the chapter.

The above is a very crude over-simplification used to clarify ideal types of political narratives. Also do not confuse small 'c' conservative with the Conservative Party; members of the Labour Party can also be *socially conservative*.

The issues of Universal Health Care (Ghebreyesus, 2017) and the need for Global Governance for Health (Ottersen et al., 2014) illustrate that both *isms* can unite on addressing health. However the unity is not to be overemphasised. Some on the *libertarian* conservative wing take the view that policy responses to the issues are far too reliant on State intervention and are thus impositions on individual liberty. The Cato Institute in the United States and the Adam Smith Institute in the UK emphasise instead much lower taxes, more reliance on private health insurance and much lower public spending. To illustrate the complexity, *The Economist* magazine (2018) which is a traditionally low tax, free market journal came out *for* Universal Health Care arguing that any infringement on individual liberty imposed by taxes for health is a price worth paying.

Two 'emergent' isms: feminism and environmentalism

The first two isms above relate to the role of the state and economics with social elements to them. Feminism and environmentalism have long histories but our two main political parties in the past have not emphasised either.

It is the case that these two 'isms' are *also* not monoliths; there are huge variances within both which at times are so far apart so as to make classification under one term problematic. Again, the following are 'ideal types'.

Feminism

Feminism is about equality of opportunity for women and about challenging current socio-political structures to address 'women's issues' such as the gender pay gap, parental leave and child care. It is also about challenging assumptions about the proper role women should play in society. More recently, high profile campaigns such as #MeToo and the 'everyday sexism' website challenge male sexual violence, sexually predatory behaviour and a sense of sexual entitlement. They point out that women should not have to defend their choice of clothes; it is for men to change their behaviour. When it comes to gender pay gaps at work, they challenge (often male) narratives that argue that the gap results from women choosing not to take on high stress, high pay jobs. They argue instead that it is structural issues like lack of parental leave, poor child care and lack of male role modelling that excludes men from caring roles. In healthcare, feminist narratives focus on the invisibility and undervaluing of care work and the structural barriers and low pay that exist for women in employment. They highlight how in both medicine and nursing, men dominate the higher consultant and managerial positions. They also highlight that the often unpaid caring burden falls upon women. Austerity policies, it is argued (MacDonald, 2018), also disproportionately affect women due to cuts in public services and female dominated public sector jobs.

In this context the narrative of the 6Cs can potentially be seen as too narrow. Produced in the wake of high profile scandals and failures within the profession, they are intended to act as an expression of the values-base for nursing, helping to ensure excellent levels of care that puts patients at the heart of everything nurses do. In this respect they can be seen as a helpful articulation of the values that many nurses will recognise and associate with, but as a response to previous instances of poor care they only present a partial picture; the 6Cs do not consider the impact of structural problems such as poor skill mix, lack of training, poor staff/patient ratios and bullying management styles focused on financial targets. Nurses, in being asked to be caring and compassionate (arguably seen as 'feminine traits'), are being positioned into 'character-based moral work' (Traynor, 2014) as a response to poor care rather than as advocates challenging policy and managerial decision making as part of their political activity (Goodman, 2016a and b).

See Finlayson, L (2016) *An Introduction to Feminism.* Cambridge: Cambridge University Press.

Environmentalism

Environmentalism is based upon the need for humanity to protect the physical environment as a fundamental basis for human health as well as being *a good thing in itself* regardless of humanity. Advocates have long pointed out issues around air pollution, deforestation, soil erosion and desertification. Barton and Grant's (2006) health map illustrate that Climate Stability, Biodiversity and the Global Ecosystem are foundational determinants of health. Lang and Rayner (2012) argue for a new paradigm in public health called 'Planetary Health' as an attempt to get health professionals talking about health from a much wider perspective than just the provision of health services such as hospitals and clinics.

Nurses who understand the sustainability agenda can challenge and assist employers in developing a sustainable NHS. They are well placed to identify sustainability problems such as the use of non-renewable products and develop sustainable solutions in clinical practice (see: NHS SDU **www.sduhealth.org.uk**). Unless nurses understand the issues they cannot advocate or speak out on these wider policy initiatives (Goodman, 2016a and b).

In both of the above isms, we argue that knowledge and understanding of their concepts and theories will give nurses a new language to talk about health and workplace practices that a purely biomedical discourse lacks. It helps to redefine clinical practice, to expand it from just the acquisition of *psychomotor* skills such as injections, towards more *cognitive* work in knowing what health is based upon and in *affective* work in developing more empathy towards each other and the environment.

See: Griffiths, J, Rao, M, Adshead, F and Thorpe, A (2009) *The Health Practitioner's Guide to Climate Change: Diagnosis and cure.* London: Earthscan.

To understand why we agree or not with party positions, we need to understand our 'moral intuitions' (Haidt, 2012) and our often unconscious narratives or 'frames' (Lakoff, 2014). The following section deals with that explanation in more detail.

This is really important to grasp because it helps us to understand why we differ so much in both the analysis of the problems we face and the solutions we might want to see.

For some, legal abortion is not the biggest social issue; for others it strikes at the heart of their morality. For others, social inequality is a good thing, and can never be got rid of, while for others there is the moral requirement to take action on the 'social determinants of health to close the gaps in social and health inequalities'.

Your professional communication and interpersonal relationships will draw from these moral positions.

Developing your political views: moral intuitions and frames

Jonathan Haidt (2012) argues we all have our often deeply held and unconscious 'moral intuitions'. Perhaps they include the need for '*care/preventing harm*' or for '*the sanctity of life*'. He suggests that when confronted with an issue, e.g. abortion, we quickly develop 'post hoc' rationalisations *based on our intuitions* when making an argument for or against. The moral intuitions came first; rationalisations come second.

Haidt's 6 Moral Foundations (**www.moralfoundations.org**):

1. Care/Harm.
2. Fairness/Cheating
3. Loyalty/Betrayal
4. Authority/Subversion
5. Sanctity/Degradation
6. Liberty/Oppression

Haidt argues that the 'Left' are rooted far more in, and value, the 'Care/Harm' and 'Fairness/Cheating' foundations. These two are often the only ones important to them.

Conservatives and the 'Right' however are also rooted in and value 'Authority/Subversion', 'Loyalty/Betrayal', 'Sanctity/Degradation' and 'Liberty/Oppression' foundations.

Consider the degree to which arguments against euthanasia, or assisted suicide, are rooted in deeply held and perhaps unexamined 'sanctity of life' morality, which then seeks post hoc rationalisations such as, 'It's the thin end of the wedge' or 'It betrays trust in doctors'. 'Sanctity' came first, the rationalisations came second. 'Sanctity' is triggered by the abortion issue. 'Abortion' transgresses the morality of the sanctity of life for 'pro-lifers'. The morality of care/harm or fairness for 'pro-choice' overrides sanctity. That is why anti-abortionists show pictures of foetuses to demonstrate in graphic detail the 'pro-life' story while pro-choice advocates will focus on telling stories on women's rights over their own bodies.

Haidt argues that our moral foundations bind us together in groups and blind us to the positions taken by others. Once you have staked out your moral positions, you engage in rationalisations to defend them. These are then often presented as objective, reasoned arguments rather than 'gut' morality ('because it is ... I dunno ... just right!').

However, if we add 'thoughtlessness', i.e. the use of cliché, convention, jargon and insider talk (Minnich, 2017) to our deeply held, unconscious, assumed and unexamined moral intuitions, we have a potent mix and an explanation for why emotional appeals in political language are so powerful. This is because stories, e.g. 'take back control' or 'for the many, not the few', trigger the deeper moral intuitions.

Narratives also have huge power because they relate to much deeper moral intuitions. This is a source of disagreement between people because they do not recognise the other person's moral intuitions or recognise that they are valid as 'morality blinds and binds', and thus they use different stories or narrative frames to argue out their positions. This is why political communication is often characterised by binary and opposing positions with very little in common. It is why they quickly become emotional.

Strict Father, Nurturing Parent: Lakoff's frames

Some of us are for: capital punishment, capping welfare and cutting social security, a strong military and intervention using force if necessary, to secure the nation's interests abroad. We may feel that for health, we should learn to take responsibility and pay for services only when we need them. Protecting people from their own poor lifestyle choices encourages 'moral hazard', in which people disregard consequences because they are protected from them, often by insurance or the NHS. The nanny state is too intrusive, should be made redundant and taxes should be 'relieved' or cut to the bone.

Much of this political positioning is down to our *moral intuitions and values* rather than as a result of rational fact and argument, which as Haidt suggests comes *afterwards*.

George Lakoff (2004, 2014) in *Don't Think of an Elephant* and *The Political Mind* attempts to describe the link between our values, what they are based in, and our political views.

To do that we have to go back to the beginning of our experiences as human beings and that means our experiences in a 'Family'. Lakoff argues that the family provides us with at least two experiences which then act as unconscious metaphors for life:

1. The Strict Father.
2. The Nurturing Parent.

These two models of family life provide us with 'frames' which are *mental structures that shape the way we see the world* (Lakoff, 2004). To over-simplify perhaps, this is to say that we all hold both frames, strict father – nurturing parent, in our heads but one may be more dominant than the other. We then approach political and social life and use these frames to explain and give meaning to what we are experiencing and to what we value.

Right, Authoritarian social conservatives tend to have a 'strict father' frame. Left, Libertarian social socialists tend to have a 'nurturing parent' frame. Thus, issues such as health behaviour and funding will be seen by referring back to those frames, and in so doing we will use particular language such as 'striver v skiver' and invoke values that accord with those frames to explain and gain meaning for issues such as 'social security'.

A frame is unconscious, part of our brain structure, and is not invoked *explicitly* in political discussions.

When using the language that arises from this frame, the frame is invoked and rein-forced. Lakoff argues that conservatives know this, and hence do not rely on reason or facts to make their case – they invoke the language of the frame and talk about their values, e.g. 'tax is theft'.

When former Health Secretary Andrew Lansley talked about the 'responsibility' deal he was invoking the 'strict father' requirement for *all of us* to exercise internal disci-pline towards our health, reinforcing the idea that we should learn to act in ways that are healthy and should learn to avoid 'feel good' but unhealthy lifestyles. If we fail to do so we should be 'punished' by experiencing the consequences of our actions. The father's (State's) job is *not* to pick up the pieces afterwards. Corporations should be *encouraged* to support us in our actions but not be *forced* to do so because in the end, it is in our own hands to choose the right path.

Let's visit 'strict father' assumptions as they apply to health; we suggest that this is the dominant narrative found in popular culture and media:

1. The world is a dangerous place and always will be, because evil exists: 'Evil' in this sense is the existence of dangerous substances such as alcohol, tobacco or illegal drugs; or it is sexual desire, lust and promiscuity resulting in STIs; or high sugar, high calorie foodstuffs. These things are 'evil' and pose a threat to our health.

2. The world is hard and difficult because it is competitive: Living healthily is tough, requires discipline and application above the norm of 'soft' living. If we don't work hard we will not get the rewards of, for example, access to gyms, or good expensive healthy food.

3. There will always be winners and losers: In health terms, this may be that we are born with good or bad genes that map out for us from birth our health pathways. Poor choices of lifestyle will always be with us. Inequality will always be with us, and it is often useless to prevent it.

4. There are absolute right and wrongs: Smoking is wrong, drinking to excess is wrong, unprotected teenage sex is wrong, illegal drug taking is wrong ... we know all of this. 'Just say No'.

5. Children are born bad, in that they only want to do that which feels good rather than that which is right: Adults act like children when they overindulge on fatty sweet foods that they know are bad for them, when they smoke knowing it kills and when they get drunk. They have not learned to discipline themselves and are acting out on 'feel good' emotions.

6. Children therefore have to be made to do the right thing: Adults however, who have not learned to do the right thing, have no internal discipline and should therefore bear the consequences of their actions. The obese are lazy and morally weak, who should just eat less and exercise more. They were not made to do the right thing and have learned unhealthy behaviours. Smokers, drinkers and drug takers should just take responsibility for their actions. Ill health that arises not from behaviour but from 'genes' or 'chance' invokes no moral opprobrium or blame and therefore health services should be provided. Illness that arises from poor choices and behaviours should really be addressed and paid for by those who make those wrong choices. Alcoholism, drug addiction, STIs and to a lesser extent diabetes as a result of obesity, or lung cancer and vascular disease from continued smoking, should attract moral judgement and justified stigma.

Activity 11.4 Critical reflection

Note down and provide examples of the degree to which you agree or disagree with the 'Strict Father' frame's assumptions.

How do you think this informs your attitudes to health behaviours and healthcare policy?

Do the same exercise for the 'Nurturing Parent' frame.

There is some brief answer guidance available at the end of the chapter.

The 'strict father' knows that adults must bear responsibility, and are no longer entitled to his protection as they should have learned right from wrong. The NHS therefore should not be there to put right the consequences of poor behaviour. Private health insurance, in this frame, ensures that the 'irresponsible' pay for their actions, or failing to take out a policy means they should properly forego treatment.

> *The 'nurturant parent' model, on the other hand, is rooted in the values of empathy and mutual responsibility. This model is gender neutral, and understands the role of parents as nurturing the inherent 'goodness' within their children through providing protection, showing them how to lead a fulfilled life, and teaching them how to empathise and care for others.*

> (Mariel Angus, 2009: **www.cpj.ca/models-morality-strict-father-and -nurturant-parent**)

As you read the next sections, think about how these family metaphors, or 'frames', might underpin opinions and attitudes towards health behaviour and lifestyle advice. You might want to revisit the idea of 'Discourse' discussed in the last chapter and Sandra Carlisle's outline of the 'Moral Underclass Discourse'. We suggest that the 'strict father' metaphor is the frame that underpins it. You might want to critically reflect on newspaper front pages and the frames they use.

Frames are important because they direct us into taking decisions about what healthcare should be, especially on what we are prepared to pay for. In the next activity, however, we might need to think about the *exercise of power* and who has a strong advocacy voice in determining what service gets funded.

Haidt's theory, Lakoff's frames and Minnich's concept of thoughtlessness point to a lack of our critical self-awareness and critical reflexivity and therefore our uncritical acceptance of assumed positions which we then might cover up with what we think is a thought-through argument. Nurses should consider, in more depth, what their positions are. You may not change your mind, but at least you will know why.

Activity 11.5 Reflection

For far too long, people of all ages with mental health problems have been stigmatised and marginalised, all too often experiencing an NHS that treats their minds and bodies separately. Mental health services have been underfunded for decades, and too many people have received no help at all, leading to hundreds of thousands of lives put on hold or ruined, and thousands of tragic and unnecessary deaths.

(The opening paragraph of the 'Five Year Forward View' review of mental health services by the Mental Health Taskforce)

What this illustrates very clearly is the existence of a long-running debate over the level of funding for core aspects of the health service. You might want to read and make notes about current and past reports and news stories about mental health provision in the coming years.

Why do you think mental health services seem to be persistently under resourced? What assumptions or assumed positions might the Mental Health Taskforce be attempting to challenge within their review?

There is some brief answer guidance available at the end of the chapter.

As noted above, political language used around health includes 'taking individual responsibility for health', often a right-wing conservative position. This view supports the policy of minimal state intervention in people's choices and lives.

The next section examines this idea more fully to argue that this is an often unexamined and dominant assumption about people's behaviour, their freedom to act and the role of the State in their lives. At the extreme end of the scale it gives rise to criticisms of public health initiatives as the 'Nanny State', which sees tax as theft and thus as morally unjustified. All nurses currently have a responsibility to promote healthy lifestyles and it is important that you begin to explore the competing political viewpoints on this topic and consider your personal position in relation to them.

The 'Liberal Human Self' and the 'neoliberal' (Right, Libertarian) political project

Much thinking and literature about our responsibilities for health, and the way we discuss health matters with others, are based on assumptions of what it is to be a human being. These assumptions include the degree of freedom we have to act. For some, our 'personal agency' is the *only* foundation upon which decisions are made and action undertaken (see Chapter 10, pp186–187).

This is the **'liberal human self'** assumption (Rossiter, 2007). The 'liberal human self' is understood to be a *free, autonomous rational* being and therefore politically should have as much freedom from interference from the State as possible to take 'individual responsibility for health'.

This set of ideas locates success and failure for health outcomes *totally within the individual.* Therefore drug addiction is a self-inflicted harm and is a result of personal moral failure and nothing to do with the society one lives in. The message here is then: 'Just Say No' to drugs. One political view on this topic (Libertarianism) is to say the State has no role here, and would argue that prohibition is poor social policy and should be repealed. People should be free to do as they please as long as they don't harm others, and suffer the consequences of their own actions.

In this idea of self, we ignore or downplay notions of 'self' that might be enabled or constrained by other, often powerful, social groups such as corporations or businesses who might be tempted to put profit before public health (Freudenberg, 2014). The dismissal of social structures, of culture, of power and of discourses is why individual choice and markets are argued by libertarians, and some conservatives, to be the best way to solve problems such as alcohol misuse, substance use and obesity.

This is the extreme end of political thinking that has *some* influence in the Conservative Party. However, Theresa May has distanced herself from such ideas criticising a belief in 'untrammelled free markets' and reiterating that there is actually a role for Government. In the 2017 Conservative Party manifesto, Theresa May argued 'we believe in the good that government can do', a statement that many libertarians would shudder at. The British Conservative Party thus has a free market (small State) wing as well as those who believe in the role for the State. You will find similar differences on the role of the State in the Labour Party.

The scenario below exemplifies the belief in the individual who can and should take responsibility for health.

Scenario: Weight control

After watching the 2015 TV show 'My Fat Story', a personal fitness instructor tested her belief in individual responsibility by deliberately putting on two stone in weight and then worked to lose it. This, she said to her clients, proves that individuals are responsible wholly for their problems and the solutions are to be found within themselves. What she argued is required is persistence, drive, motivation and willpower, and perhaps a gym membership. Her attitude was that 'fat people are lazy' and 'there is no excuse for obesity. It's simple maths.'

While reading the scenario above to what extent did you find yourself agreeing or disagreeing with the fitness instructor? You might want to look up the research on willpower as a means to change and maintain behaviour. When it comes to weight loss and the significance of willpower the evidence seems to suggest that it is not actually all that powerful, argues University of Minnesota health psychologist Traci Mann (2015): *Secrets From the Eating Lab: The Science of Weight Loss, the Myth of Willpower, and Why You Should Never Diet Again.* Are you surprised by this? If so start to think about why that might be the case.

This view of self leads to an emphasis on education, information and personal responsibility because, in this view, there *is nothing else existing other than the sovereign individual* that can do the work of improving one's health.

This idea of the free 'liberal human self' is a *political project* because it fits with a much bigger political ideology: 'neoliberalism' (Gonçalves et al., 2015; Goodman, 2017). The two concepts need each other; they need to exclude ideas of the social in human affairs because once one concedes that health and illness may have something to do with the social and the political, and is not only down to irrational morally corrupt individual choices, then solutions to health and illness might also have to be social and political.

Health promotion theory, such as Beattie's model (1991) used by public health professionals, goes way beyond this simplistic 'liberal human self' approach. However, 'Health Promotion' remains political in that there is no consensus on either explanations *of* or interventions *for* health and health inequalities (Carlisle, 2001). If you are to be a politically aware practitioner it is important that you recognise these different viewpoints and how they can influence health policy formation and implementation.

Politics, public health and health inequalities: the case of obesity

The statistics on obesity rates are well published and easily accessible, especially in journals such as *The Lancet.* You could access their series of papers (2015, 2017) on 'Obesity'; just go to **www.thelancet.com** and search for obesity. The journal suggests that by 2030 almost 50% of the world's population will be overweight or obese if current rates continue. This perspective has been criticised as 'fatphobic' (Lupton, 2013) and overly medical, using the language of pandemic and 'health crisis'. For our purposes, let's accept this paradigm at face value to outline the solution put forward.

For example, the UK's Childhood Obesity Strategy (Great Britain, HM Government, 2016) refrained from restricting price cutting promotions and junk food marketing and advertising. Instead it relies on behaviour change and individually focused measures such as school activity programmes. The latter, it has been claimed, do not work (Adab et al., 2018).

Deborah Lupton's work on 'Fat Politics' (2013) criticises the *overly individualised* understanding of and responses to weight gain and reminds us to think about the social and political context. That context includes the tactics used by 'Big Food' to prevent State action on their activities, as the health organisation Vital Strategies in their report 'Fool Me Twice' argues. The food industry's messages include: 'Do not restrict individual freedom; it is up to people to show self-discipline; products are only occasional indulgences'.

Some countries have tried to tackle the industry, instead of relying on voluntary action. In Latin America, governments have forced companies to remove cartoon characters from cereal boxes, imposed junk food taxes and ordered school tuck shops to replace high salt and high sugar products with fruit and vegetables.

The argument here is that rules, regulations, laws (State Intervention) can reshape consumer perceptions and decision making, and that over time individuals come to 'construct' a self that does not include the consumption of high sugar content products.

Nurses' health messages will be partly based on what they believe to be true and what they think the role of government and individuals should be. On obesity, we suggest that an overly biomedical, mechanistic approach has come to dominate health discourse.

Hunter et al. (2009) asked why better progress has not been made to reduce obesity. One answer is that solutions (a) too often *reduce* the problem to biology: calories in must equal calories out and (b) are *mechanistic* assuming that intervention A will cause effect B: e.g. more exercise = weight loss.

The Foresight Report (2007) on obesity identified the 'obesogenic environment' which challenges the focus on individual behaviour change and simple education messages. Simple solutions (reductionist and mechanistic) such as targeting obese individuals with messages about eating less and moving more are only a small part of the solution. Foresight suggests there is no simple or single solution that works in a mechanistic cause–effect way. Policies like 'Change4Life' (**www.nhs.uk/change4life/about-change4life**) which focuses on individual lifestyle changes and behaviour changes will not be enough. 'Change4Life' and other individually focused interventions fail to engage with Foresight's 'whole systems approach'. Obesity has to be seen as a result of an interrelationship of factors, e.g. food production and processing including the use of sugar, corporate lobbying and power relationships, poverty, employment patterns and structures, transport and fast food availability. In this view, nurses giving out health behaviour change advice are unwitting participants in an *individualising* and *ineffective* health policy while at the same time letting other powerful actors, such as the food industry, off the hook.

In *Lethal but Legal*, Freudenberg (2014) argues that the most important and modifiable causes of ill health include the *triumph of a political and economic system that promotes consumption at the expense of health* (p.viii). To address issues such as global obesity requires *taking on the world's most powerful corporations and their allies*. Similarly, Stuckler and Basu (2013) point to Government policy, specifically austerity, as a danger to public health due to cuts in services. Marmot (2015) argues that inequality is a key factor for differential health outcomes. He suggests that conventional approaches that have emphasised technical solutions and changes in the behaviour of individuals (lifestyle drift) can only go so far. What is required is changing the social and political conditions so people can have control over their lives, to have the power to live as they decide.

'Lifestyle drift' (Hunter et al., 2009) is the tendency for policy initiatives, for example Foresight, to recognise the need to take action on the wider determinants of health, i.e. recognising 'upstream' public health (RCN, 2012), but which as they get implemented they drift 'downstream' (RCN, 2012) to focus on *individual lifestyle factors*. Nurses are then co-opted in implementing these downstream policies.

This is in contrast to the World Health Organization's call to 'take action on the *social* determinants of health' and the Lancet Commission's call for Global Governance for Health (Ottersen et al., 2014), both of which accept the need for State action.

Activity 11.6   Critical thinking

Consider your position on this question:

Does obesity, poverty and ill health arise from the failings of individuals or from failings of society?

- Write some first thoughts on this question and share with colleagues.
- What evidence do you have for your position? Can you refer to any?
- What should the appropriate role of the State be: Education or Intervention?

As this relies on your individual responses there is no answer at the end of the chapter.

The next section looks at the 'contextual issues' of the 'wider determinants of health' and what individual responsibility singularly fails to address or communicate to populations. In your everyday health education and health promotion activities with individuals, communities and populations, you will be discussing interventions and solutions and you will be introduced in all probability to 'wider/social determinants of health' during your education. You will also be exposed to 'lifestyle drift' solutions.

Activity 11.7   Critical thinking

See the RCN's (2012) 'Going Upstream: nursing's contribution to public health. Prevent, promote and protect.' Read the document and consider if any of it might be criticised as too 'nanny state' (Right, Libertarian) or not interventionist *enough* (Left, Authoritarian)?

There is some brief answer guidance available at the end of the chapter.

The wider determinants of health

An individual's health is determined by their biology up to a degree. However, there is a growing acceptance that health has much wider determinants that go beyond genetic inheritance.

A *macro* determinant is the political structures we all live in. This is the focus of Ottersen et al.'s (2014) outline of the need for Global Governance for Health.

WHO (2008) defines the *social* determinants of health as:

> *the conditions in which people are born, grow, live, work and age, including the health system. These circumstances are shaped by the distribution of money, power and resources at global, national and local levels. The social determinants of health are mostly responsible for health inequities – the unfair and avoidable differences in health status seen within and between countries.*

Data on health inequalities in the UK is readily available in *Fair Society Healthy Lives* (Marmot, 2010) and books such as *The Spirit Level* by Richard Wilkinson and Kate Pickett and *Inequality and the 1%* by Danny Dorling. The Public Health Observatory publishes 'Community Health Profiles' (see: Public Health England's health profiles site: **https://fingertips.phe.org.uk/profile/health-profiles**). This lists indicators of health and allows you to make comparisons between more or less deprived areas of the UK.

The wider socio-political context that impacts on global population health are outlined in the box below. When one begins to consider wider, global health issues then political issues become even more salient for discussion.

Theory summary: Global contextual factors for health

Wolfgang Streeck (2016) calls the current global order one of multi-morbidity; climate change being one of many frailties as we head towards social entropy, radical uncertainty and indeterminacy. We thus have global challenges to the social order, which have current and future impacts on health and healthcare delivery. Streeck argues that the current context is anchored in a variety of interconnected developments including rising social inequality and populist nationalism and the spectre of fascism in Europe and isolationism in the US. To that we could add continuing health inequalities, the potential for ecosystem collapse and the emergence of disruptive technologies: Automation, Artificial Intelligence and Digitalisation.

Countervailing voices paint more positive pictures: Joseph Norberg (2016) on the possibility and actuality of progress, Daniel Ben-Ami (2010) on the ability of growth-based capitalism to solve ecological problems and Stephen Pinker (2011) on reducing levels of global violence.

We suggest that these important issues are often invisible in health policy documents or in advice for, and the education of, nurses. It could be that these issues are beyond health professionals' control or remit. However, we provide them here for your critical reflection on what determines health. You might want to then think about what the appropriate response could be.

Universal healthcare, comprehensive and equitable health cover, free at the point of delivery, are not experienced equally across the globe. Health outcomes such as mortality rates, life expectancy, disability free life expectancy, the under 5 mortality rate, suicide rates, and other indicators are characterised by inequality often linked to socio-economic status (the 'social gradient') but also with gender and ethnic dimensions to them. It is true to say that great progress has been made on these indicators (see for example Hans Rosling's Gapminder website), but progress cannot be taken for granted without the political will to continue. The 'Sustainable Development Goals' also known as 'Global Goals', are ambitions to address health and social inequalities, Every health professional should be at least aware of them. See **globalgoals.org**.

It could be suggested that global health challenges and the context are immediate and dangerous. The existence of health inequalities has been known since at least the publication of the Black Report in 1980. We may wish to ask we if are acting quickly enough to deal with them, i.e. is there enough political will to address the issues?

So far we have tried to reflect on the messages we receive and communicate to individuals, communities and populations on health issues such as health inequalities and the wider determinants of health. In the next section we wish to critically reflect on how the political and institutional context shapes professional discourse and practices.

Power, policy and health outcomes: what is nursing's role?

There is perhaps a causal relationship between inequalities in health and the social, material, political and cultural inequalities of the wider determinants of health. Scambler's (2012) health assets approach argues that material health assets are paramount in determining health outcomes. His 'Greedy Bastards Hypothesis' asserts that health inequalities in Britain are first and foremost an *unintended consequence* of the 'strategic' behaviours at the core of the country's *capitalist-executive* and *power elite*.

Numerous examples can be found where corporate activities have impacted on scientific and political decision making on such issues as global warming, DDT and acid rain (Oreskes and Conway, 2010; Monbiot, 2013; Drutman, 2015). Further recent examples include the motor industry effectively lobbying for delays in implementation of new air pollution standards (Archer, 2015) or Volkswagen's use of software to cheat emissions testing in the US (*Guardian*, 2016). These examples indicate the lengths that some corporations will go to avoid the costs of dealing with environmental and health regulations (Wiegratz and Whyte, 2016).

Following Scambler's hypothesis, companies such as VW do not *intend* to increase respiratory deaths linked to air pollution, but in trying to avoid exhaust emission standards, the *consequences* of their actions can be seen to do so. The historical and current lobbying by industry linked scientists (Oreskes and Conway, 2012) to prevent legislative action (e.g. on tobacco, sugar) is a 'strategic action' that has health consequences.

The UK's Responsibility Deal (2011) argued:

> *By working in partnership, public health, commercial, and voluntary organisations can agree practical actions to secure more progress, more quickly, with less cost than legislation.*

(see: **https://responsibilitydeal.dh.gov.uk/wp-content/uploads/2012/03/
The-Public-Health-Responsibility-Deal-March-20111.pdf**)

This statement looks like a reasoned, technical, neutral and evidence-based approach, but it also fits very well with neoliberal assumptions about the proper and in their view, very limited, role of the State. Note that statements like this form part of an overall 'discourse'.

However, Hunter et al. (2009) argue:

> *The only way to achieve lasting reductions in inequality is to address society's imbalances with regard to power, income, social support and knowledge ... implement upstream policy interventions ... supported by downstream interventions.*

(Priority Public Health Conditions, Task group 8)

The profession of nursing has a history of political activism for health (Falk-Raphael, 2006). An issue for today's graduate nurses is the degree to which they are exposed to and understand discourses that go beyond individualised biomedical approaches to care so that they can continue to take their place in health advocacy and activism (Goodman, 2015; Goodman and Grant, 2017) so that we may get both a 'fair society *and* healthy lives'. The NMC (2018) have made it clear that this is an important element of the nursing role stating that nurses need to *understand the mechanisms that can be used to influence organisational change and public policy, demonstrating the development of political awareness and skills* throughout their career in order to maximise their impact.

Activity 11.8   Research and evidence-based practice

1. Go to the Fairer Society Healthy Lives website (**www.instituteofhealthequity. org**). Find the executive summary of *The Marmot Review* (2010).

    - What are the key messages of the review? Explain in your own words.
    - How many policy objectives are there?
    - What are the key points from each?
    - What sort of data is this based on?

2. Go to Marmot Indicators for local authorities (**www.gov.uk/government/ collections/phe-london-advice-support-and-services**).

    (a) Choose South West in 'select your region', then select 'Cornwall'.

    (b) Do the same for Northeast and Newcastle, London and Hackney, London and Kensington and Chelsea.

    (c) Open the pdfs. What are you looking at? Compare the data sets.

There are no answers on this activity at the end of the chapter.

That nursing work is embedded in a political context but without always being explicitly so, is exemplified by the at times uncritical use of certain terms. This language of nursing includes words such as 'Accountability' and of course more recently the language of the 6Cs. The ongoing cases of care failures are the context for this language use. However, emphasising 'individual nursing accountability' has been a core feature in nursing for decades. The word 'care' itself is arguably one of the most often used words in the nursing profession's lexicon.

We invite you to think about why this is. Given the current context which involves arguments around the sustainability of health and social care funding, poor quality care of frail older people and those with learning disabilities, does the focus on the need for 'accountable care-giving' run into the problem of overly individualising the solution for care failures which actually result from much bigger political decision-making? It might seem that individualising the problem of care-giving by asking nurses to improve on care and compassion, mirrors the individualising of responsibility for health. What if it is the case that there are structural and political reasons, as well for poor quality care provision, and not just uncaring staff (Goodman, 2014; Goodman, 2016b)?

To be clear, we are not suggesting here that nurses should not be held accountable for their individual actions. The *Code* exists for very explicit and important reasons and you must constantly bear in mind that failing to comply with it can result in you being referred to an NMC Fitness to Practise tribunal and potentially struck off the register.

That being said, we also need to think what 'accountability' might mean in situations in which the carrying out of the normal functions of one's job result in very negative experiences for people. We need to think whether the standards and conditions of employment based in health and social policy are such that to comply with those standards means poor service.

It is perfectly possible to meet one's accountability to the employer but to miss completely one's accountability to people. Activity 11.9 asks you to consider this question. If there was a conflict of interest between your duty to your employer or your duty to your patients, what decision will you make? This is a political decision as well as a professional and ethical one.

Activity 11.9   Critical thinking

The 2016 Parliamentary Ombudsman report of unsafe discharges of people from hospital illustrates care failures that arise not because of deliberate malice or abuse, but because of systematic and probably everyday practices that result in poor assessment and communication between staff. Nurses have to liaise with doctors and other health professionals while also working within hospital management guidance. Conflicts of interest can arise and priorities misalign that result in unsafe discharge. Read the nine cases studies very carefully. Consider what your course of action would be when disagreement arises about discharge followed by an actual discharge that you are not happy with. Think very carefully about to whom you are accountable and to whom you will seek advice and guidance.

See: The Parliamentary and Health Service Ombudsman 'A report into investigations of unsafe discharge from hospital' (2016). **www. ombudsman.org.uk/**

A further example is illustrated by the case of a patient with MS who had a decision to reduce a 24-hour care package reduced to 12 hours against the patient's GP's advice. The patient was assessed by an employee of Atos who had been contracted by the Department of Work and Pensions to assess the needs of patients receiving a Personal Independence payment. To whom was the assessor being accountable in practice: the Department of Work and Pensions or the patient with MS? This could be an example of complying with one's job specifications and yet be involved in inhumane practice. The Atos assessor in doing the job perhaps far too well was complying with policy, but to what end? It is not always clear what qualifications Atos assessors have, but we do know that registered nurses work as Atos assessors. How does this reconcile with the values articulated within the 6Cs?

This is not a new issue, and it requires individuals to be critically aware of how the institutional context can directly affect both the nature of communication and inter-personal relationships one is developing. Activity 11.10 asks you to consider how the concept of Institutional Violence may exist in which professionals might consider that they are 'just doing my job' expressed through certain discourses and narratives.

Activity 11.10   Institutional violence: 'I'm just doing my job'

Read the following two definitions of violence:

1. Johan Galtung (1969) argued: *Violence is present when human beings are being influenced so that their actual somatic and mental realisations are below their potential realisations.* He further argued:

   - *Violence is a phenomenon which reduces a person's potential for performance. A distinction must be made between violence and force, since the former breeds negative results, while this is not necessarily so in the case of the latter. This is an important option, because many people consider that violence may have both positive and negative results.*
   - *Violence should be objectively measured according to its results, not in a subjective manner. Indicators could be suicide, mental illness, mortality and morbidity rates, hunger, and poverty.*

2. Felipe MacGregor and Marcial Rubio refer back to Galtung and provide their own definition of violence:

   A physical, biological or spiritual pressure, directly or indirectly exercised by a person on someone else, which, when exceeding a certain threshold, reduces or annuls that person's potential for performance, both at an individual and group level, in the society in which this takes place.

Reflect on whether any healthcare context can exert indirect physical or spiritual pressure.

Some may doubt the existence of institutional violence, perhaps arguing that only human beings can directly inflict pain. The work of Erving Goffman and his idea of the 'total institution' may still be pertinent here (Davies, 1989; Goodman, 2013). Criticism of the idea of structural or institutional violence, and the denial thereof, may focus on the need for an actor; an actor who can then be held liable for such action. Personal or direct violence is a violence in which an aggressor can be identified, face to face, whereby the victim can recognise a guilty person through direct confrontation. However, the focus on violent or abusive individuals may obscure that they might work within organisational forms and within institutional arrangements that are themselves violent.

Following the work Goffman in the 1960s, Johan Galtung (1969) wrote of *structural* violence; a violence in which some social structure or social institution causes harm by preventing people from meeting basic needs. This is a model of violence that goes beyond notions that focus only on individual agency.

Gregg Barak (2003) argues:

> *Like interpersonal forms of violence, institutional forms include physically or emotionally abusive acts. However, institutional forms of violence are usually, but not always, impersonal: that is to say, almost any person from the designated group of victims will do.*
>
> (p77)

Barak goes on:

> *Moreover, abuses or assaults that are practiced by corporate bodies – groups, organisations, or even a single individual on behalf of others – include those forms of violence that over time have become institutionalized … These forms of violence may be expressed directly against particular victims by individuals and groups or indirectly against entire groups of people by capricious policies and procedures carried out by people 'doing their jobs', differentiated only by a myriad of rationales.*
>
> (p77)

People 'doing their jobs' using policies, routine, custom and practice, thoughtlessness, banality and cliché to justify their actions may unwittingly be inflicting a form of violence upon vulnerable groups of people. For an example, see Death by Indifference (Mencap, 2007) and The Learning Disability Mortality Review 2016–2017 (LeDeR, 2018). We suggest that you keep a critical eye on the literature reporting and analysing care for vulnerable groups of people to consider where accountability for their experiences is to be found.

Chapter summary

We began by outlining what politics might mean for nurses, emphasising that it is not to be bound by 'party politics', rather that it embraces many topic areas including health inequalities. We outlined common 'isms' and suggested by the use of the political compass that political positions have both economic and social dimensions to them. Moral Foundations Theory and Frames were introduced to suggest our political views arise not always from clear analytical thinking, but from deeper intuitive moral responses and narratives. This was followed by a discussion exploring a particular view of what we are – the 'liberal human self' – to suggest that it is a flawed model explaining who we are and what we do. It fails to take into account society and powerful agents and vested interests. It also supports overly simplistic approaches to public health, particularly obesity. We suggested this fits well into a particular political philosophy – neoliberalism (Gonçalves et al., 2015; Goodman, 2017) – which overemphasises the role of the individual in taking responsibility for health and because it considers state intervention to be less than helpful, it shifts the responsibility towards individuals and families. It also fails to account for ideas of the complexity of our social and political relations as in, for example, the obesogenic environment. We briefly outlined some key ideas around health inequalities and the wider determinants of health to suggest that avoidable illness and deaths are related to social and political actions. We suggested that this also happens at the local level even when we may be implementing agreed policy. Finally we suggested that our actions and justifications can operate within institutional or structural violence which we might be blind to. This context radically forms the communication and interpersonal skills and relationships we then engage in.

Activities: brief outline answers

Activity 11.4: Critical reflection (p219)

Note down and provide examples of the degree to which you agree or disagree with the Strict Father frame's assumptions.

How do you think this informs your attitudes to health behaviours and healthcare policy?

Do the same exercise for the 'Nurturing Parent' frame.

A Nurturing Parent frame may see that obesity arises from influences other than moral weakness. It would point to the myriad opportunities provided each day to overeat, and that it is in some people's interest to encourage overeating. Punishment is thus not an appropriate a strategy. Instead, one would seek to provide people with strategies to avoid overeating while also calling for protection from the predatory actions of those who profit from obesity.

Activity 11.5: Reflection (p220)

Why do you think mental health services seem to be persistently under resourced? What assumptions or assumed positions might the Mental Health Taskforce be attempting to challenge within their review?

One answer is the dominance of the biomedical model and easily identifiable physical illness having a historical grip on NHS resources. The invisible nature of much of psychological distress and the lack of treatment options and conflicting paradigms for care have prevented a robust national approach. Mental illness has had a historical stigma and fear attached to it, and is little understood by the public.

Activity 11.7: Critical thinking (p225)

On page 15 of the document is an example of prevention: a stop smoking service in secondary care. It can be seen as 'nannying' smokers in hospital through assessment of smoking status and offering support to smokers in *every clinical contact*, to improve uptake to effective forms of support either via referral or medication. This applies subtle pressures to people who freely choose to smoke. It can also be seen as not interventionist enough by not classifying tobacco in the same way as other drugs are classified as A, B or C.

Further reading

'Fool Me Twice: An NCD Advocacy report' argues that food, soda and alcohol companies are promoting products that undermine health and wellbeing using tactics and strategies comparable to the tobacco industry from two decades ago. The report is available here: **www.vitalstrategies.org/publications/fool-twice-ncd-advocacy-report/**

Haidt, J (2012) *The Righteous Mind: Why good people are divided by politics and religion*. London: Penguin.

This book, by a psychologist, argues that we have moral intuitions that come before reasoned argument, and explores the problems this can cause.

Lupton, D (2013a) *Fat Politics: Collected writings*. Sydney: University of Sydney. Available at **http://hdl.handle.net/2123/9021**.

Lupton, D (2013b) *Revolting Bodies: The pedagogy of disgust in public health campaigns*. Sydney Health & Society Group Working Paper No. 4. Sydney: Sydney Health & Society Group. Available at **http://hdl.handle.net/2123/9110**.

Lupton, D (2017) Vitalities and visceralities: Alternative body/food politics in new digital media. In: *Alternative Food Politics: From the margins to the mainstream*, edited by Michelle Phillipov and Katherine Kirkwood. London: Routledge, forthcoming.

Smith, K, Hill, S and Bambra, C (2016) *Health Inequalities: Critical perspectives*. Oxford: Oxford University Press.

A good, explanatory textbook on health inequalities.

Traynor, M (2013) *Nursing in Context: Policy, politics, profession*. Basingstoke: Palgrave Macmillan.

Examines the policy and political context of nursing.

Useful websites

Which UK party might you identify with?
uk.isidewith.com/political-quiz

Why people disagree about politics:
www.yourmorals.org/

The Equality Trust:
www.equalitytrust.org.uk

The Adam Smith Institute: a UK Free Market Neoliberal think tank:
www.adamsmith.org

Glossary

autonomous reflexivity: Margaret Archer's concept of our thinking that is oriented to ourselves; self-referential thinking in deciding what course of action to take.

biomedical model: a model employing the principles of biology, biochemistry, physiology and other basic sciences to solve problems in clinical medicine.

blip culture: contemporary healthcare cultures where there is only time for brief interpersonal exchanges between nurses and their patients.

communication: the reciprocal and effective process in which messages are sent and received between two or more people.

communicative reflexivity: Margaret Archer's concept of our thinking that is orientated towards others, considering what other people think before a course of action is undertaken.

confirmation bias: A cognitive bias in which we attend to evidence that confirms our theory and disregards evidence that contradicts our theory.

control: central to good mental health; people who function well at the level of their mental health experience high levels of subjective control; the opposite is true for those who experience mental health difficulties.

counterculture: the consciously held negative views of a minority of individuals against the dominant culture.

critical realism: social theory associated with Roy Bhaskar and Margaret Archer which argues for the necessity of ontology. This means being able to speak and understand 'being' apart from human thought and language. It argues that things exists apart from our experience and knowledge of those things.

critical reflexivity: the active practice of personal awareness that goes beyond personal introspection to take into account the social and political contexts and drivers of professional practice.

critical theory: an approach to understanding society by exploring culture, economics, politics and power relationships.

cultural relativism: a culture or civilisation where there is the belief that concepts such as right and wrong, goodness and badness, or truth and falsehood are not absolute but change from culture to culture, and situation to situation.

culture: the dominant mores, habits and beliefs of a group of people, usually united by their ethnic, social, sexual or other orientation.

culture-centrism: talking, thinking and behaving from a position where one's own culture and cultural identity are assumed to be the 'correct' one, from which other cultures and cultural identities are judged to be lacking, deviant or incorrect.

discourse: an institutionalised pattern of speech which reflects power through the use of knowledge, thereby creating our worlds.

discrimination: the conscious or unconscious negative views of individuals, on the basis of their ethnicity, sexual orientation or lifestyle.

empathy: the ability to be attuned, and respond appropriately, to the inner experience and distress of patients.

ethnicity: ethnic affiliation or distinctiveness.

ethnocentricity: the 'taken-for-granted' views held by members of a society, which, they believe, apply globally.

ethnocentrism: a belief in, or assumption of, the superiority of the social or cultural group that a person belongs to.

evidence-based practice: the combination of the best available scientific evidence and theories informing safe and effective interpersonal communication in nursing.

existential–phenomenological: personal experience and responsibility of the individual, who is seen as a free agent, and the doctrine that all knowledge comes from perceptions of what is sensed by the individual.

experiential learning: learning that is derived from or relating to experience, as opposed to other methods of acquiring knowledge.

fundamental attribution error: a cognitive bias in which we ignore situational factors for someone's behaviour while over-confidently attributing that behaviour to their fundamental character.

fractured reflexivity: Archer's concept of our thinking that is so disoriented it provides little guide to action.

gestalt: a set of things, such as a person's thoughts and experiences, considered as a whole and regarded as amounting to more than the sum of its parts; a set of items or things that are regarded as a whole.

governmentality: the process by which power is exercised in a diffuse way so that we come to govern ourselves and each other, without the need to refer to formal authority.

healthy relating: the use of good communication and interpersonal skills between nurses, their colleagues and their patients; good communication is respectful, non-exploitative, non-judgemental and formal rather than casual.

helping relationship: a relationship between a nurse and someone in the nurse's care which proves of value to the latter, in regard to helping the person positively move forward in life.

humanistic approach: implies that individuals can solve their own problems independent of cultural and organisational constraints.

immigration: coming into a foreign country to settle there.

individualism: from an 'individualistic' perspective, people are assumed to have the power to find their own solutions to their problems, independent of cultural or organisational constraining factors.

informatics: the science of processing data for storage and retrieval; information science.

interpersonal skills: skills that are exhibited when nurses demonstrate their abilities to use evidence-based, and theory-based, styles of communication with their patients and colleagues.

liberal human self: a rational, free thinking self who exists independently from society.

lifestyle drift: tendency for policy initiatives to recognise the need to take action on the wider determinants of health but which, as they get implemented, drifts to focus on individual lifestyle factors.

loss: a feature of the subjective experience of depression or low mood.

metacognitive: refers to the idea of 'thinking about thinking'; this means, in practice, thinking about the ways in which you, as a nurse, and your patients think about the ways in which you and they think.

meta reflexivity: Archer's concept of thinking about one's own thinking, especially considering values and whether action possible.

migration: going from one place to another.

moral practice: in nursing, refers to the respectful treatment of a patient as a fully human being, rather than an object or an 'it'.

nurse-focused: refers to the defensive ways in which nurses often communicate with their patients; these forms of communication are often guarded, withdrawn and distancing, leaving patients feeling more anxious and lonely than they otherwise might be.

ontology: the enquiry into meanings and categories of existence or being.

prejudice: bigoted views held by members of one culture against members of another.

professional artistry: embodied skilled practice that proceeds from the tacit knowledge resources held by experienced professionals.

professional relationship: the connection between two or more people or groups and their involvement with one another, especially with regard to the way they behave towards and feel about one another, which is focused around an occupation as a paid job rather than a hobby.

rationalisation: finding reasons to explain or justify one's actions.

reflective writing: writing that is characteristic of and expresses contemplative, analytical and careful thoughts.

Rogerian principles: refers to the position that the 'core conditions' of Rogerian-informed interpersonal communication are both necessary and sufficient; these conditions are 'non-judgementalism', 'unconditional positive regard' and 'genuineness'.

schemas: psychological templates, or mental structures, that we all develop to make sense of the world; they help us develop general expectations about ourselves, others, social roles and events, and how to behave in specific situations.

self-awareness: our knowledge about ourselves, our motivations, and how these translate into our behaviours.

self-esteem: individuals' subjective experience of the overall effectiveness they possess in the conduct of their lives; low self-esteem, therefore, indicates a lowered experience of such effectiveness.

social relationship: the connection between two or more people or groups and their involvement with one another, especially with regard to the way they behave towards and feel about one another, focused around human society and how it is organised.

social rules: authoritative principles set forth to guide behaviour or action and that relate to the connection between two or more people or groups and their involvement with one another, especially with regard to the way they behave towards and feel about one another.

social thinking: use of the mind to form thoughts, opinions, judgements and conclusions about the ways in which people in groups behave and interact.

suffering: individuals who are suffering exhibit high levels of distress in relation to their physical or mental anguish.

technical rationality: an approach to practice that matches problems occurring in the professional world with discrete solutions, which arguably takes insufficient account of the complexities of practice.

theory of mind: the ways in which all human beings make inferences and guesses about what they think is going through the minds of others and what informs their behaviour.

therapeutic relationship: relates to or involves activities carried out to maintain or improve somebody's health within the professional relationship defined above.

Transactional Analysis: a psychodynamic theory which emphasises the role of internal consciousness and emotion expressed as 'ego states' for communicating.

transcultural: a sophisticated awareness of the beliefs, feelings and behaviours of members of cultures other than one's own.

unhealthy relating: an abandonment of the moral, psychological and empathic basis for caring, interpersonal communication; organisational environments will contribute to the shaping of healthy and unhealthy relating between nurses and patients.

References

Abramovitz, M and Zelnick, J (2010) Double jeopardy: the impact of neoliberalism on care workers in the United States and South Africa. *International Journal of Health Services*, *40*(1): 97–117.

Action on Elder Abuse (2017) *What is Elder Abuse?* Available at: www.elderabuse.org.uk.

Adab, P, Pallan, M, Lancashire, E, et al. (2018) Effectiveness of a childhood obesity prevention programme delivered through schools, targeting 6 and 7 year olds: cluster randomised controlled trial (WAVES study). *BMJ, 360*: K211.

Adorno, T and Horkheimer, M (1944) *Dialectic of Enlightenment as Philosophische Fragmente*. New York: Social Studies Association.

Allport, G (1954) *The Nature of Prejudice*. Boston, MA: Addison-Wesley.

Alvesson, M and Spicer, A (2012) A stupidity-based theory of organizations. *Journal of Management Studies, 49*(7): 1194–1120.

Anderson, N, Calvillo, ER and Fongwa, MN (2007) Community-based approaches to strengthen cultural competency in nursing education. *Journal of Transcultural Nursing, 18*: 49–59.

Aramburu Alegria, C (2011) Transgender identity and health care: implications for psychosocial and physical evaluation. *Journal of the American Academy of Nurse Practitioners, 23*: 175–182.

Archer, G (2015) Governments double and delay air pollution limits for diesel cars. Available at: www.transportenvironment.org/press/governments-double-and-delay-air-pollution-limits-diesel-cars.

Archer, M (2003) *Structure, Agency and the Internal Conversation*. Cambridge: Cambridge University Press.

Archer, M (2013) Reflexivity. Sociopedia.*isa*. Available at: www.sagepub.net/isa/resources/pdf/Reflexivity2013.pdf.

Armstrong, AE (2006) Towards a strong virtue ethics for nursing practice. *Nursing Philosophy, 7*: 110–124.

Arnold, E and Boggs, KU (2006) *Interpersonal Relationships: Professional communication skills for nurses*, 4th edn. London: Elsevier.

Arnold, E and Boggs, KU (2015) *Interpersonal Relationships: Professional communication skills for nurses*, 7th edn. Philadelphia, PA: WB Saunders.

Arntz, A and Van Gerderen, H (2009) *Schema Therapy for Borderline Personality Disorder.* Chichester: Wiley-Blackwell.

Aston, M, Price, S, Kirk, S and Penney, T (2011) More than meets the eye: feminist poststructuralism as a lens towards understanding obesity. *Journal of Advanced Nursing,* *68*(5): 1187–1194.

Augoustinos, M, Walker, I and Donaghue, N (2014) *Social Cognition: An integrated introduction,* 3rd edn. London: Sage.

Bach, S (2004) *Psychological Care in Community Nursing: A phenomenological investigation.* PhD thesis, University of Manchester.

Baker, C (2013) Introduction. In: Baker, C, Shaw, C and Biley, F (eds). *Our Encounters with Self-Harm.* Ross-on-Wye: PCCS Books.

Baker, C, Shaw, C and Biley, F (eds) (2013) *Our Encounters with Self-Harm.* Ross-on-Wye: PCCS Books.

Balzer-Riley, J (2004) *Communication in Nursing.* Mosby, MO: Mosby/Elsevier.

Banister, P and Kagan, C (1985) The need for research into interpersonal skills. In: Kagan, C (ed.) *Interpersonal Skills in Nursing: Research and applications.* London: Croom Helm, pp44–60.

Barak, G (2003) *Violence and Nonviolence.* Los Angeles: Sage.

Baron-Cohen, S (2003) *The Essential Difference: Men, women and the extreme male brain.* London: Basic Books.

Barton, H and Grant, M (2006) A health map for the local human habitat. *Journal of the Royal Society for the Promotion of Health, 126*(6): 252–261.

Baxter, C (2000) Antiracist practice: achieving competency and maintaining professional standards. In: Thompson, T and Mathias, P (eds). *Lyttle's Mental Health and Disorder.* Edinburgh: Bailliere Tindall.

Beattie, A. (1991) Chapter 7. In: Gabe, J, Calnan, M and Bury, M. *Sociology of the Health Service.* London: Routledge.

Belbin, M (1981) *Management Teams.* Oxford: Butterworth-Heinemann.

Ben-Ami, D (2010) *Ferrari's for All: In defence of economic progress.* Bristol: Policy Press.

Bendall, E (1976) Learning for reality. *Journal of Advanced Nursing, 1*: 3–9.

Bendall, E (2006) 30th anniversary commentary on Bendall E. 1976 'Learning for reality'. *Journal of Advanced Nursing,* 30th anniversary issue.

Benner, P (1982) From novice to expert. *American Journal of Nursing, 82*(3): 402–407.

Benner, PD (2000) *From Novice to Expert: Excellence and power in clinical nursing practice, commemorative edition.* Upper Saddle River, NJ: Prentice Hall.

Benner, P and Wrubel, J (1988) The primacy of caring. *American Journal of Nursing, 88*(8): 1073–1075.

Benner, P, Tanner, C and Chesla, C (1996) *Expertise in Nursing Practice: Caring, clinical judgement, and ethics*. New York: Springer.

Bhaskar, R (1975 [1997]) *A Realist Theory of Science*, 2nd edn. London: Verso.

Birch, K (2015) How to think like a neoliberal. *Discover Society*. Issue 22. Available at: http://theconversation.com/how-neoliberalisms-moral-order-feeds-fraud-and-corruption-60946.

Bowlby, J (1988) *A Secure Base: Clinical applications of attachment theory*. London: Routledge.

Brown, B, Crawford, P and Carter, R (2006) *Evidence-Based Health Communication*. Maidenhead: Open University Press and McGraw-Hill Education.

Brown, LP (2011) Revisiting our roots: caring in nursing curriculum design. *Nurse Education in Practice, 11*(6): 360–364.

Bruff, I (2017) *Authoritarian Neoliberalism and the Myth of Free Markets*. Available at: http://ppesydney.net/authoritarian-neoliberalism-myth-free-markets/

Brykczynska, G (1997) A brief overview of the epistemology of caring. In: Brykczynska, G (ed.) *Caring: The compassion and wisdom of nursing*. London: Arnold/Allen Lane, pp1–9.

Buber, M (1958) *I and Thou*, 2nd edn. New York: Charles Scribner.

Burnard, P (1996) *Acquiring Interpersonal Skills: A handbook of experiential learning for health professionals*, 2nd edn. London: Chapman and Hall.

Butland, B, Jebb, S, Kopelman, P, McPherson, K, Thomas, S, Mardell, J and Parry, V (2007) *Foresight. Tacking Obesities: Future choices*. London: Government Office for Science.

Byrd, ME, Costello, J, Gremel, K, Blanchette, MS and Malloy, TE (2012) Political astuteness of Baccalaureate nursing students following an active learning experience in health policy. *Public Health Nursing, 29*(5): 433–443.

Canales, MK (2010) Othering: difference understand? A 10-year analysis and critique of the nursing literature. *Advances in Nursing Science, 33*(1): 15–34.

Carlisle, S (2001) Inequalities in health: contested explanations, shifting discourses and ambiguous polices. *Critical Public Health, 11*(3): 267–281.

Carnegie, E and Kiger, A (2009) Being and doing politics: an outdated model or 21st century reality. *Journal of Advanced Nursing, 65*(9): 1976–1984.

Cave, T (2010) Nurses for reform. *BMJ, 340*:1371.

Chaffee, MW, Mason, DJ and Leavitt, JK (2012) A framework for action in policy and politics. In: Mason, DJ, Leavitt, JK and Chaffee, MW (eds). *Policy and Politics in Nursing and Healthcare*, 6th edn. St Louis: Elsevier Saunders.

Charlton, CR, Dearing, KS, Berry, JA and Johnson, MJ (2008) Nurse practitioners' communication styles and their impact on patient outcomes: an integrated literature review. *Journal of the American Academy of Nurse Practitioners, 20*: 382–388.

Charon, R (2006) *Narrative Medicine: Honoring the stories of illness*. Oxford and New York: Oxford University Press.

Cioffi, J (2006) Culturally diverse patient–nurse interactions on acute care wards. *International Journal of Nursing Practice*, 12(6): 319–325.

Clarke, JB and Wheeler, SJ (1992) A view of the phenomenon of caring in nursing practice. *Journal of Advanced Nursing*, 17: 1283–1290.

Clarke, S, Davies, H, Jenney, M, Glaser, A and Eiser, C (2005) Parental communication and children's behaviour following diagnosis of childhood leukaemia. *Psycho-Oncology*, 14(4): 274–281.

Clay, M and Povey, R (1983) Moral reasoning and the student nurse. *Journal of Advanced Nursing*, 8: 297–302.

Corbally, M and Grant, A (2016) Narrative competence: a neglected area in undergraduate curricula. *Nurse Education Today*, 36: 7–9.

Corrie, S, Townend, M and Cockx, A (2016) *Assessment and Case Formulation in Cognitive Behavioural Therapy*, 2nd edn. London: Sage.

Cortis, JD (1993) Transcultural nursing: appropriateness for Britain. *Journal of Advances in Health and Nursing Care*, 12(4): 67–77.

Crawford, P (2014) *Florence Nightingale carried the lamp but modern nurses carry the can.* Available at: http://theconversation.com/florence-nightingale-carried-the-lamp-but-modern-nurses-carry-the-can-25114.

Cunningham, G and Kitson, A (2000a) An evaluation of the RCN clinical leadership development programme: Part 1. *Nursing Standard*, 15(12): 34–37.

Cunningham, G and Kitson, A (2000b) An evaluation of the RCN clinical leadership development programme: Part 2. *Nursing Standard*, 15(13): 34–40.

Curtis, K (2013) 21st century challenges faced by nursing faculty in educating for compassionate practice: embodied interpretations of phenomenological data. *Nurse Education Today*, 33(7): 746–750.

Davidson, C (1985) The theoretical antecedents to interpersonal skills training. In: Kagan, C (ed.) *Interpersonal Skills in Nursing: Research and applications*. London: Croom Helm, pp22–43.

Davidson, L, Sharp, M and Halford, J (2010) Antisocial and borderline personality disorders. In: Grant, A, Townend, M, Mulhern, R and Short, N (eds). *Cognitive Behavioural Therapy in Mental Health Care*, 2nd edn. London: Sage.

Davies, B and Harre, R (1990) Positioning: the discursive production of selves. *Journal of the Theory of Social Behaviour*, 20: 43–65.

Davies, C (1989) Goffman's concept of the total institution: criticisms and revisions. *Human Studies*, 12(1/2): 77–95.

Department for Children, Schools and Families (2004) *The Children Act 2004*. London: Stationery Office.

Department of Health (DH) (2003) *Getting the Right Start: The National Service Framework for Children, Young People and Maternity Services – Standards for Hospitals Services.* London: Stationery Office.

Department of Health (DH) (2004) *Getting Over the Wall: How the NHS is improving the patient's experience.* London: Department of Health.

Department of Health (DH) (2006) *The Expert Patients Programme.* Available at: www.dh.gov.uk.

Department of Health (DH) (2010) *Advanced Level Nursing: A position statement.* London: Department of Health.

Department of Health (DH) (2011) *Liberating the NHS: An information revolution – a consultation document.* London: Department of Health.

Department of Health (DH) (2012) *Transforming Care: A national response to Winterbourne View Hospital Department of Health review – final report.* London: Department of Health.

Department of Health (DH) (2013) *Report of the Mid-Staffordshire NHS Foundation Trust Public Inquiry.* London: The Stationery Office.

Dixon, J and Levine, M (2012) *Beyond Prejudice: Extending the social psychology of conflict, inequality and social change.* Cambridge: Cambridge University Press.

Dorling, D (2015) *Unequal Health: The scandal of our times.* Bristol: Policy Press.

Drach-Zahavy, A and Hadid, N (2015) Nursing handovers as resilient points of care: linking handover strategies to treatment errors in the patient care in the following shift. *Journal of Advanced Nursing, 71*(5): 1135–1145.

Drury, J (2003) Adolescent communication with adults in authority. *Journal of Language and Social Psychology, 22*(1): 66–73.

Drury, J (2015) The nature of adolescence and its family, societal, community, cultural, and developmental challenges. In: Crome, I and Williams, R (eds). *Substance Misuse and Young People.* London: Hodder & Stoughton.

Drury, J, Catan, L and Dennison, C (1998) Young people's communication difficulties: experiences with employers and family adults. *Journal of Youth Studies, 1*(3): 245–257.

Drury, J, Cocking, C and Reicher, S (2009) Everyone for themselves? A comparative study of crowd solidarity among emergency survivors. *British Journal of Social Psychology, 48*: 487–506.

Drutman, L (2015) *The Business of America is Lobbying: How corporations became politicised and politics became more corporate.* Oxford: Oxford University Press.

Dunhill, l and Williams, D (2016) Mackey tells Trusts to curb staff growth. *Health Service Journal.* Available at: www.hsj.co.uk/topics/workforce/exclusive-mackey-tells-trusts-to-curb-clinical-staff-growth/7006372.article

Edmonstone, J (2009) Clinical leadership: the elephant in the room. *International Journal of Health Planning Management, 24*(4): 290–305.

Edmonstone, J (2014) Whither the elephant?: the continuing development of clinical leadership in the UK National Health Services. *International Journal of Health Planning and Management, 29*(3): 280–291.

Egan, G (2014) *The Skilled Helper: A problem management approach to helping,* 10th edn. Belmont, CA: Brooks Cole.

Eisenstein, C (2013) *The More Beautiful World Our Hearts Know is Possible.* Berkeley: North Atlantic Books.

Ellaway, R, Coral, J, Topps, D and Topps, M (2015) Exploring digital professionalism. *Medical Teaching, 37*(9): 844–849.

Erikson, K (2002) Caring science in a new key. *Nursing Science Quarterly, 15*(1): 61–65.

European Union (EU) (2004) *Enabling Good Health for All: A reflection process for a new EU strategy.* Available at: http://ec.europa.eu/health/ph_overview/Documents/byrne_reflection_en.pdf.

Evans, D, Coutsaftiki, D and Fathers, P (2014) *Health Promotion and Public Health for Nursing Students,* 2nd edn. London: Sage Publications.

Falk, JH (2014) Lifelong learning. In: *Encyclopaedia of Science Education.* Netherlands: Springer, pp1–2.

Falk-Rafael, A (2006) Globalization and global health: toward nursing praxis in the global community. *Advances in Nursing Science, 29*(1): 2–14.

Favretto, AR and Zaltron, F (2013) Children, parents and paediatricians: adequate parenting representations in the therapeutic relation. *Quaderni ACP, 20:* 109–112.

Fennell, M (1999) *Overcoming Low Self-esteem: A self-help guide using cognitive behavioural techniques.* London: Robinson.

Finlayson, L (2016) *An Introduction to Feminism.* Cambridge: Cambridge University Press.

Fiske, ST and Taylor, SE (1991) *Social Cognition,* 2nd edn. New York: McGraw-Hill.

Fitzsimmons, P (1999) Managerialism and education. In: Peters, P, et al. (eds). *The Encyclopedia of Educational Philosophy and Theory.* London: Taylor and Francis.

Fortman, J (2003) Adolescent language and communication from an intergroup perspective. *Journal of Language and Social Psychology, 22*(1): 104–111.

Foucault, M (1963) *The Birth of the Clinic: An archaeology of medical perception.* London: Routledge.

Foucault, M (1969) *The Archaeology of Knowledge.* London: Routledge.

Foucault, M (1975) *Discipline and Punish: The birth of the prison.* London: Routledge.

Francis, R (2013) *Report of the Mid Staffordshire NHS Foundation Trust Public Inquiry.* Available at: www.midstaffspublicinquiry.com/report.

Frankfurt, H (2005) *On Bullshit.* Available at: www.stoa.org.uk/topics/bullshit/pdf/on-bullshit.pdf.

Freshwater, D and Rolfe, G (2001) Critical reflexivity: a politically and ethically engaged research method for nursing. *NT Research*, 6(1): 526–537.

Freudenberg, N (2014) *Lethal but Legal.* New York: Oxford University Press.

Frew, E and Hollingsworth, B (2017) *How financial incentives could help tackle Britain's childhood obesity problem. The Conversation.* March 2nd. Available at: https://theconversation.com/how-financial-incentives-could-help-tackle-britains-childhood-obesity-problem-71355.

Frost, PJ, Dutton, JE, Worlen, MC and Wilson, A (2000) Narratives of compassion in organizations. In: Fineman, S (ed.) *Emotion in Organizations*, 2nd edn. London: Sage.

Fyffe, T (2009) Nursing shaping and influencing health and social care policy. *Journal of Nursing Management*, 17(6): 698–706.

Gerrish, K, Husband, C and Mackenzie, J (1996) *Nursing for a Multi-ethnic Society.* Buckingham: Open University Press.

Ghebreyesus, TA (2017) All roads lead to universal health coverage. *The Lancet*, 5(9).

Gilbert, P (2009) *The Compassionate Mind.* London: Constable.

Gilbert, P and Leahy, R (eds) (2007) *The Therapeutic Relationship in the Cognitive Behavioural Psychotherapies.* Hove: Routledge.

Goffman, E (1959) *The Presentation of Self in Everyday Life.* London: Penguin.

Goffman, E (1961) Asylums. *Essays on the Social Situation of Mental Patients and Other Inmates.* New York: First Anchor Books.

Goffman, E (1972) *Strategic Interaction.* New York: Ballantine.

Goleman, D (2006) *Social Intelligence: The new science of human relationships.* London: Hutchinson.

Gonçalves, F, Oliviera-Souza, S, Gollner-Zeitoune, R, et al. (2015) Impacts of neoliberalism on hospital nursing work. *Texto contexto-enferm*, 24(3): 646–653.

Goodman, B (2003) Ms B and legal competence: examining the role of nurses in difficult ethico-legal decision making. *Nursing in Critical Care*, 8(2): 78–83.

Goodman, B (2004) Ms B and legal competence: interprofessional collaboration and nurse autonomy. *Nursing in Critical Care*, 9(6): 271–276.

Goodman, B (2011) The one dimensional state of (UK) nurse education. *Nurse Education Today*, 31(8): 725–726.

Goodman, B (2013) Erving Goffman and the total institution. *Nurse Education Today*, 33(2): 81–82.

Goodman, B (2014) Risk rationality and learning for compassionate care: the link between management practices and the 'lifeworld' of nursing. *Nurse Education Today*, 34(9): 1265–1268.

Goodman, B (2015a) Caring in an uncaring society. *Journal of Clinical Nursing*, 24 (13–14): 1741–1742.

Goodman, B (2015b) *Psychology and Sociology in Nursing*. London: Sage.

Goodman, B (2016a) Lying to ourselves: rationality, critical reflexivity and the moral order as structured agency. *Nurse Education Today. Nursing Philosophy, 17*(3): 211–221.

Goodman, B (2016b) The missing two Cs – commodity and critique: obscuring the political economy of the gift of nursing. *Journal of Research in Nursing, 21*(4): 325–335.

Goodman, B (2017a) *Neoliberalism: Rhetoric and reality*. Available at: www.bennygoodman. co.uk/neoliberalism-rhetoric-and-reality/

Goodman, B (2017b) *Alpha males, psychopaths and Greedy Bastards*. Available at: www. bennygoodman.co.uk/alpha-males-psychopaths-and-greedy-bastards/

Goodman, B and East, L (2014) The sustainability lens: a framework for nurse education that is fit for the future. *Nurse Education Today, 34*(1): 100–103.

Goodman, B and Grant, A (2017) The case of the Trump regime: the need for resistance in international nurse education. *Nurse Education Today, 52*: 53–56.

GOV.UK. (2013) *Case Study: The Expert Patients Programme*. Available at: www.gov.uk/ government/case-studies/the-expert-patients-programme.

Grant, A (2000) Clinical supervision and organisational power: a qualitative study. *Mental Health and Learning Disabilities Care, 31*(12): 398–401.

Grant, A (2010a) A brief history of cognitive behavioural therapy. In: Grant, A (ed.) *Cognitive Behavioural Interventions for Mental Health Practitioners*. Exeter: Learning Matters.

Grant, A (2010b) Helping people with borderline personality disorder. In: Grant, A (ed.) *Cognitive Behavioural Interventions for Mental Health Practitioners*. Exeter: Learning Matters.

Grant, A (2010c) Writing the reflexive self: an autoethnography of alcoholism and the impact of psychotherapy culture. *Journal of Psychiatric and Mental Health Nursing, 17*: 577–582.

Grant, A (ed.) (2010d) *Cognitive Behavioural Interventions for Mental Health Practitioners*. Exeter: Learning Matters.

Grant, A (2013) Writing teaching and survival in mental health: a discordant quintet for one. In: Short, NP, Turner, L and Grant, A (eds). *Contemporary British Autoethnography*. Rotterdam: Sense Publishers, pp33–48.

Grant, A (2014a) Breaking the grip: a critical insider account of representational practices in cognitive behavioural psychotherapy and mental health nursing. In: Zeeman, L, Aranda, K and Grant, A (eds). *Queering Health: Critical challenges to normative health and healthcare*. Ross-on-Wye: PCCS Books, pp116–133.

Grant, A (2014b) Neoliberal higher education and nursing scholarship: power, subjectification, threats and resistance. *Nurse Education Today, 34*: 1280–1282.

Grant, A (2015) Demedicalising misery: welcoming the human paradigm in mental health nurse education. *Nurse Education Today, 35*: e50–e53.

Grant, A (2016a) Living my narrative: storying dishonesty and deception in mental health nursing. *Nursing Philosophy, 17*: 194–201.

Grant, A (2016b) Storying the world: a posthumanist critique of phenomenological–humanist representational practices in mental health nurse qualitative inquiry. *Nursing Philosophy, 17*: 290–297.

Grant, A and Barlow, A (2016) The practitioner/survivor hybrid: an emerging anti-stigmatising resource in mental health care. *Mental Health Practice, 20*(1): 33–37.

Grant, A and Leigh-Phippard, H (2014) Troubling the normative mental health recovery project: the silent resistance of a disappearing doctor. In: Zeeman, L, Aranda, K and Grant, A (eds). *Queering Health: Critical challenges to normative health and healthcare.* Ross-on-Wye: PCCS Books, pp100–115.

Grant A and Radcliffe, M (2015) Resisting technical rationality in mental health nurse higher education: a duoethnography. *The Qualitative Report (TQR), 20*(6) Article 6: 815–825.

Grant, A, Mills, J, Mulhern, R and Short, N (2004) *Cognitive Behavioural Therapy in Mental Health Care.* London: Sage.

Grant, A, Townend, M, Mills, J and Cockx, A (2008) *Assessment and Case Formulation in Cognitive Behavioural Therapy.* London: Sage.

Grant, A, Townend, M, Mulhern, R and Short, N (eds). (2010) *Cognitive Behavioural Therapy in Mental Health Care,* 2nd edn. London: Sage.

Grant, A, Biley, F and Walker, H (eds) (2011) *Our Encounters with Madness.* Ross-on-Wye: PCCS Books.

Grant, A, Haire, J, Biley, F and Stone, B (eds) (2013) *Our Encounters with Suicide.* Ross-on-Wye: PCCS Books.

Grant, A, Leigh-Phippard, H and Short, N (2014) Re-storying narrative identity: a dialogical study of mental health recovery and survival. *Journal of Psychiatric and Mental Health Nursing, 22*(4): 1187–1194.

Grant A, Leigh-Phippard, H and Short, NP (2015a) Re-storying narrative identity: a dialogical study of mental health recovery and survival. *Journal of Psychiatric and Mental Health Nursing, 22*: 278–286.

Grant, A, Zeeman, L and Aranda, K (2015b) Queering the relationship between evidence-based mental health and psychiatric diagnosis: some implications for international mental health nurse curricular development. *Nurse Education Today,* e18–e20.

Grant, A, Naish, J and Zeeman, L (2016) Depathologising sexualities in mental health services. *Mental Health Practice, 19*(7): 26–31.

Greenberg, LS (2007) Emotion in the therapeutic relationship in emotion-focused therapy. In: Gilbert, P and Leahy, R (eds). *The Therapeutic Relationship in the Cognitive Behavioural Psychotherapies.* Hove: Routledge.

Greenhalgh, T and Hurwitz, B (1999) Why study narrative. *BMJ, 318*: 48–50.

Griffiths, J, Rao, M, Adshead, F and Thorpe, A (2009) *The Health Practitioner's Guide to Climate Change: Diagnosis and cure.* London: Earthscan.

Guardian, The (2016) *The Volkswagen emission scandal explained.* Available at: www.theguardian.com/business/ng-interactive/2015/sep/23/volkswagen-emissions-scandal-explained-diesel-cars.

Haidt, J (2012) *The Righteous Mind: Why good people are divided by politics and religion.* London: Penguin.

Hall, ET (1966) *The Hidden Dimension.* New York: Doubleday.

Hall, S (2011) The neoliberal revolution. *Cultural Studies*, 25(6): 705–728.

Hallström, I and Runneson, I (2001) Needs of parents of hospitalized children. *Theoria: Journal of Nursing Theory*, 10: 20–27.

Ham, C (2014) *Reforming the NHS from Within: Beyond hierarchy, inspection and markets.* London: The Kings Fund.

Hargie, O (ed.) (2006) *The Handbook of Communication Skills*, 3rd edn. London: Routledge.

Hargie, O (2011) *Skilled Interpersonal Communication: Research, theory and practice*, 5th edn. London and New York: Routledge.

Hargie, O (2016) *Skilled Interpersonal Communication: Research, theory and practice*, 6th edn. London: Routledge.

Hartrick, G (1997) Relational capacity: the foundation for interpersonal nursing practice. *Journal of Advanced Nursing*, 26: 523–528.

Hayes, SC and Smith, S (2005) *Get Out of Your Mind and Into Your Life: The new acceptance and commitment therapy.* Oakland, CA: New Harbinger.

Hebdidge, D (1979) *Subculture: The meaning of style.* London: Routledge.

Helman, C (2001) *Culture, Health and Illness*, 4th edn. London: Edwin Arnold.

Henderson, IW (1967) Psychological care of patients with malignant disease. *Applied Therapy*, 9(10): 827–832.

Hillman, A, Tadd, W, Calnan, S, Calnan, M, Bayer, A and Read, S (2013) Risk, governance and the experience of care. *Sociology of Health and Illness*, 35(6): 939–955.

Hogg, MA and Vaughan, GM (2011) *Social Psychology*, 6th edn. Harlow: Pearson Education.

Holmes, D, Murray, S, Perron, A, et al. (2006) Deconstructing the evidence-based discourse in health sciences: truth, power and fascism. *International Journal of Evidence Based Healthcare*, 4(3): 180–186.

Holstein, JA and Gubrium, JF (2000) *The Self We Live By: Narrative identity in a postmodern world.* New York: Oxford University Press.

Holyoake, D (2011) Is the doctor nurse game being played? *Nursing Times*, 107(43).

Honey, P and Mumford, A (1992) *The Manual of Learning Styles.* Maidenhead: Peter Honey.

Hood, C (1991) A public management for all seasons. *Public Administration, 69*(1): 3–19.

Horkheimer, M (1982) *Critical Theory.* New York: Continuum.

Horton, E (2007) Neoliberalism and the Australian Healthcare System (factory). *Proceedings 2007, Conference of the Philsophy of Education Society of Australasia.* Wellington. Available at: http://eprints.qut.edu.au/14444/1/14444.pdf.

Howard, A (2001) Fallacies and realities of self. *Counselling and Psychotherapy Journal, 12*(4): 19–23.

Howe, D (2013) *Empathy: What it is and why it matters.* Basingstoke: Palgrave Macmillan.

Hudson, C, McDonald, B, Hudson, J, Tran, D and Boodhwani, B (2015) Impact of anesthetic handover on mortality and morbidity in cardiac surgery: a cohort study. *Journal of Cardiothoracic and Vascular Anesthesia, 29*(1): 11–16.

Hunter, D, Popay J, Tannahill C, Whitehead, M and Elson, T (2009) *Learning Lessons from the Past: Shaping a Different Future written by the Marmot Review Working Committee 3 – Crosscutting sub group report.* (November 2009). Available at: www.instituteofhealthequity.org/projects/the-marmot-review-working-committee-3-report.

The Independent, 17 Nov 2016. *Brexit: EU nurses are 'suffering racist abuse and heading home',a Parliamentary inquiry is told.* Available at: www.independent.co.uk/news/uk/politics/brexit-eu-nurses-are-suffering-racist-abuse-and-heading-home-a-parliamentary-inquiry-is-told-a7423611.html.

Jasper, M (1996) The first year as a staff nurse: the experiences of a first cohort of Project 2000 nurses. *Journal of Advanced Nursing, 24*: 779–790.

Jenerette, C and Brewer, C (2011) Situation, Background, Assessment, and Recommendation (SBAR) may benefit individuals who frequent emergency departments: adults with sickle cell disease. *Journal of Emergency Nursing, 37*(6): 559–561.

Jones, A (2007) Putting practice into teaching: an exploratory study of nursing undergraduates' interpersonal skills and the effects of using empirical data as a teaching and learning resource. *Journal of Clinical Nursing, 16*: 2297–2307.

Jones, LJ (1994) *The Social Context of Health and Health Care.* Basingstoke: Macmillan.

Jones, R (2016) On course to tweet. *Nursing Standard (Royal College of Nursing), 30*(27): 26–27.

Jones, RB, Ashurst, EJ and Trappes-Lomax, T (2015) Searching for a sustainable process of service user and health professional online discussions to facilitate the implementation of e-health. *Health Informatics Journal, 22*(4): 948–961.

Jones, R, Kelsey, J, Nelmes, P, Chinn, N, Chinn, T and Proctor-Childs, T (2016) Introducing Twitter as an assessed component of the undergraduate nursing curriculum: case study. *Journal of Advanced Nursing, 72*(7): 1638–1653.

Kahneman, D (2011) *Thinking Fast and Slow*. London: Penguin.

Katzenbach, JR and Smith, DK (1993) The discipline of teams. *Harvard Business Review, 71* (March–April): 111–146.

Kennett, C and Payne, M (2009) Palliative care patients' experiences of healthcare treatment. *International Journal of Social Welfare, 19*(3): 262–271.

Kemppainen, V, Tossavainen, K and Turunen, H (2012) Nurses' roles in health promotion practice: an integrative review. *Health Promotion, 28*(4): 490–501.

Kitson, AL (2003) A comparative analysis of lay-caring and professional (nursing) caring relationships. *International Journal of Nursing Studies, 40*(5): 503–510.

Kitwood, T (1997) *Dementia Reconsidered: The person comes first*. Buckingham: Open University Press.

Kohut, H (1984) *How Does Analysis Cure?* Chicago: University of Chicago Press.

Kolb, DA (2000) *Facilitator's Guide to Learning*. Boston, MA: Hay/McBer.

Kolb, DA and Fry, D (1975) Towards an applied theory of experiential learning. In: Cooper, CL (ed.) *Theories of Group Processes*. Chichester: Wiley.

Kouzes, J and Posner, B (2011) *The Five Practices of Exemplary Leadership*. San Francisco: Pffeifer.

Kyle, TV (1995) The concept of caring: a review of the literature. *Journal of Advanced Nursing, 21*: 506–514.

Laing, RD (1960) *The Divided Self: An existential study in sanity and madness*. London: Penguin.

Lakoff, G (2004/2014) *Don't think of an elephant! Know your values and frame the debate*. Chelsea Green: White River Junction.

The Lancet (2017) Syndemics: health in context. *The Lancet, 389*,10072: 881. Available at: http://thelancet.com/journals/lancet/article/PIIS0140-6736(17)30640-2/fulltext.

Lang, K, Neil, J, Wright, J, et al. (2013) Qualitative investigation of barriers to accessing care by people who inject drugs in Saskatoon, Canada: perspectives of service providers. *Substance Abuse Treatment, Prevention and Policy*, 8.35. Available at: https://doi. org/10.1186/1747-597X-8-35.

Lang, T and Rayner, G (2012) Ecological public health: the 21st century's big idea? *BMJ, 345*: e5466.

Lauder, W, Reynolds, W, Smith, A and Sharkey, S (2002) A comparison of therapeutic commitment, role support, role competency and empathy in three cohorts of nursing students. *Journal of Psychiatric and Mental Health Nursing, 9*: 483–491.

Lea, A, Watson, R and Deary, IJ (1998) Caring in nursing: a multivariate analysis. *Journal of Advanced Nursing, 28*: 662–671.

LeDeR (2018) *The Learning Disabilities Mortality Review Annual Report 2017*. Bristol: University of Bristol.

Leigh-Phippard H and Grant A (2017) Freedom and consent. In: Chambers M (ed.) *Psychiatric and Mental Health Nursing: The craft of care*, 3rd edn. London and New York: Routledge, pp191–200.

Leininger, MM (1981) The phenomenon of caring: importance, research questions and theoretical considerations. In: Leininger, MM (ed.) *Caring, and Essential Human Need*. Detroit, MI: Wayne State University Press.

Leininger, MM (1984) *Care: The essence of nursing and health*. Detroit, MI: Wayne State University Press.

Leininger, MM (1997) Transcultural nursing research to nursing education and practice: 40 years. *Image: Journal of Nursing Scholarship, 29*(4): 341–347.

Lencioni, P (2002) *The Five Dysfunctions of a Team*. San Francisco: Jossey-Bass.

Lencioni, P (2017) Accountability in team culture: a path to increased performance. Available at: https://learningwire.crossknowledge.com/accountability-culture.

Levetown, M (2008) Communicating with children and families: from everyday interactions to skill in conveying distressing information. *American Academy of Pediatrics, 121*(5): 1441–1460.

Levine, M and Crowther, S (2008) The responsive bystander: how social group membership and group size can encourage as well as inhibit bystander intervention. *Journal of Personality and Social Psychology, 95*(6): 1429–1439.

Lewis, CC, Pantell, RH and Sharp, L (1991) Increasing patient knowledge, satisfaction and involvement: randomised trial of a communication intervention. *Pediatrics, 88*(2): 351–358.

Long, A (ed.) (1999) *Interaction for Practice in Community Nursing*. Basingstoke: Macmillan.

Lorig, K, Ritter, P, Dost, A, Plant, K, Laurent, D and McNeil, I (2008) The expert patients programme online, a 1-year study of an Internet-based self-management programme for people with long-term conditions. *Chronic Illness, 4*(4): 247–256.

Lovering, S (2006) Cultural attitudes and beliefs about pain. *Journal of Transcultural Nursing, 17*(4): 389–395.

Lupton, D (2013) *Fat*. London: Routledge.

Maben, JA, Latter, SB and Clark, JM (2006) The theory–practice gap: impact of professional–bureaucratic work conflict on newly qualified nurses. *Journal of Advanced Nursing, 55*(4): 465–477.

Maben, J, Latter, S and Macleod Clark, J (2007a) The challenges of maintaining ideals and standards in professional practice from a longitudinal study. *Nursing Inquiry, 14*(2): 99–113.

Maben, JA, Latter, SB and Clark, JM (2007b) The sustainability of ideals, values and the nursing mandate: evidence from a longitudinal qualitative study. *Nursing Inquiry, 14*: 99–113.

McCabe, C and Timmins, F (2006) *Communication Skills for Nursing Practice.* London: Palgrave Macmillan.

McCabe, C and Timmins, F (2013) *Communication Skills for Nursing Practice,* 2nd edn. London: Palgrave Macmillan.

McCarthy-Jones, S (2017) The concept of schizophrenia is coming to an end – here's why. *The Conversation.* 24 August. Available at: https://theconversation.com/the-concept-of-schizophrenia-is-coming-to-an-end-heres-why-82775.

MacDonald, Ellie Mae (2018) *The gendered impact of austerity: cuts are widening the poverty gap between women and men. British Politics and Policy at LSE* (10 Jan 2018). Blog Entry.

MacGregor, F and Rubio, M (1994) Remythologizations of power and identity: nationalism and violence in Sri Lanka. In Rupesinghe, K and Rubio, M (eds) *The Culture of Violence.* Tokyo: United Nations University Press.

MacLeod Clark, J (1985) The development of research in interpersonal skills. In: Kagan, C (ed.) *Interpersonal Skills in Nursing: Research and applications.* London: Croom Helm, pp9–21.

McMahon, R (1993) Therapeutic nursing: theory, issues and practice. In: McMahon, R and Pearson, A (eds). *Nursing as Therapy,* 2nd edn. London: Chapman Hall.

MacNaught, A (1994) A discriminating service: the socioeconomic and scientific roots of racial discrimination in the National Health Service. *Journal of Inter-Professional Care, 8*: 143–149.

Macpherson of Cluny, W (Chair) (1999) *The Stephen Lawrence Inquiry.* London: Stationery Office.

McSherry, R, Pearce, P, Grimwood, K and McSherry, W (2012) The pivotal role of nurse managers, leaders and educators in enabling excellence in nursing care. *Journal of Nursing Management, 20*(1): 7–19.

Mann, Traci (2015) *Secrets from the Eating Lab: The science of weight loss, the myth of willpower, and why you should never diet again.* New York: Harper Wave.

Marcuse, H (1964) *One Dimensional Man.* London. Routledge.

Marmor, T (2005) *Fads, Fallacies and Foolishness in Medical Care Management and Policy: The rhetoric and reality of managerialism.* Rock Carling Fellowship. London: Nuffield Trust and The Stationary Office.

Marmor, T (2007) *Fads, Fallacies and Foolishness in Medical Care.* Singapore: World Scientific Publishing Co.

Marmot, M (2010) *Fair Society, Healthy Lives: Strategic review of health inequalities in England post 2010.* Available at: www.instituteofhealthequity.org/projects/fair-society-healthy-lives-the-marmot-review.

Melia, K (1984) Student nurses' construction of occupational socialisation. *Sociology of Health and Illness, 2*(2): 132–151.

Mencap (2007) *Death by Indifference.* London: Mencap.

Menzies Lyth, I (1988) *Containing Anxiety in Institutions: Selected essays.* London: Free Association Books.

Meyerson, DE (2002) If emotions were honoured: a cultural analysis. In: Fineman, S (ed.) *Emotion in Organizations,* 2nd edn. London: Sage.

Minnich, E (2017) *The Evil of Banality: On the life and death importance of thinking.* Rowman and New York: Littlefield.

Miranda, R and Andersen, SM (2007) The therapeutic relationship: implications from social cognition and transference. In: Gilbert, P and Leahy, RL (eds). *The Therapeutic Relationship in the Cognitive Behavioural Psychotherapies.* Hove: Routledge.

Mitchell, G and Agnelli, J (2015) Person-centred care for people with dementia: Kitwood reconsidered. *Nursing Standard, 30*(7): 46–50.

Monbiot, G. (2013) *It's business that really rules us now.* Available at: www.theguardian. com/commentisfree/2013/nov/11/business-rules-lobbying-corporate-interests.

Morgan, G (2006) Organization as psychic prison. In: Morgan, G. *Images of Organization,* updated edition. London: Sage Publications.

Morrison, P and Burnard, P (1991) *Caring and Communicating: The interpersonal relationship in nursing.* Basingstoke: Macmillan.

Morse, JM, Bottorff, J, Neander, W and Solberg, S (1991) Comparative analysis of conceptualisations and theories of caring. *Image: Journal of Nursing Scholarship, 23*(2): 119–126.

Morse, JM, Bottorff, J, Anderson, G, O'Brien, B and Solberg, S (1992) Beyond empathy: expanding expressing of caring. *Journal of Advanced Nursing, 17*: 809–821.

Muir Gray, JA (1997) *Evidence-Based Healthcare: How to make health policy and management decisions.* New York: Churchill-Livingstone.

Narayanasamy, A and White, E (2005) A review of transcultural nursing. *Nurse Education Today, 25*: 102–111.

National Audit Office (2018) The adult social care workforce. London: NAO. Available at: www. nao.org.uk/wp-content/uploads/2018/02/The-adult-social-care-workforce-in-England.pdf

National Health Service (NHS) Modernisation Agency (2003) *Essence of Care, Guidance and New Communication Benchmarks.* London: Department of Health.

National Health Service (NHS) (2009) *Using Mobile Phones in Hospital.* Available at: http:// webarchive.nationalarchives.gov.uk/20130107105354/www.dh.gov.uk/prod_consum_ dh/groups/dh_digitalassets/@dh/@en/documents/digitalasset/dh_092812.pdf.

National Health Service (NHS) (2014) *Change4Life.* Available at: www.england.nhs.uk/ wp-content/uploads/2014/10/5yfv-web.pdf.

National Health Service England (NHSE) (2014) Five Year Forward View. *NHSE.* London. Available at: www.england.nhs.uk/wp-content/uploads/2014/10/5yfv-web.pdf.

Newell, R and Gournay, K (eds) (2000) *Mental Health Nursing: An evidence-based approach.* London: Churchill- Livingstone.

NHS England (2014a) *Accessible Information.* Available at: www.england.nhs.uk/ourwork/patients/accessibleinfo-2.

NHS England (2014b) *Patient OnLine.* Available at: www.england.nhs.uk/ourwork/pe/patient-online.

Norberg, J (2016) *Progress: 10 reasons to look forward to the future.* London: Oneworld.

Norcross, JC (2011) *Psychotherapy Relationships That Work: Therapist contributions and responsiveness to patients,* 2nd edn. New York: Oxford University Press.

Nursing and Midwifery Council (NMC) (2004a) *Standards of Proficiency for Pre-registration Nursing Education.* London: NMC.

Nursing and Midwifery Council (NMC) (2004b) *The NMC Code of Professional Conduct: Standards for conduct, performance and ethics.* London: NMC.

Nursing and Midwifery Council (NMC) (2008) *The Code: Standards of conduct, performance and ethics for nurses and midwives.* London: NMC.

Nursing and Midwifery Council (NMC) (2010) *Standards for Pre-registration Nursing Education.* London: NMC.

Nursing and Midwifery Council (2018) *Future Nurse: Standards of Proficiency for Registered Nurses.* London: NMC.

Nussbaum, JF, Pecchioni, LL, Robinson, JD and Thompson, TL (2000) *Communication and Aging,* 2nd edn. Mahwah, NJ: Lawrence Erlbaum Associates.

Oakley, J (2000) Gender based barriers to senior management positions: understanding the scarcity of female CEOs *Journal of Business Ethics, 27*(4): 321–334.

O'Keefe-McCarthy, S (2008) Women's experiences of cardiac pain: a review of the literature. *Canadian Journal of Cardiovascular Nursing, 18*(3): 18–25.

Oliver, M (1990) *The Politics of Disablement.* London: Macmillan.

O'Neill, O (2002) *A Question of Trust: The BBC Reith Lectures 2002.* New York: Cambridge University Press.

Open Learn (2017) The Open University 'Issues in Complementary and Alternative Medicine'. Available at: www.open.edu/openlearn/health-sports-psychology/health/health-studies/issues-complementary-and-alternative-medicine/content-section-0.

Oreskes, N and Conway, E (2010) *Merchants of Doubt.* London: Bloomsbury.

Ottersen, O, Dasgupta, J, Blouin, C, et al. (2014) The Lancet–University of Oslo Commission on Global Governance for Health. *The Political Origins of Health Inequity: Prospects for Change. The Lancet,* 383: 630–667.

Ousey, K and Johnson, M (2007) Being a real nurse: concepts of caring and culture in the clinical areas. *Nurse Education in Practice, 7*(3): 150–155.

Padesky, C (1991) Schema as self-prejudice. Reprinted from the *International Cognitive Therapy Newsletter, 6*: 6–7 (1990).

Parfitt, B (1998) *Working Across Culture: A study of expatriate nurses working in developing countries in primary health care.* Aldershot: Ashage.

Parsons, T (1951) *The Social System.* Glencoe, IL: The Free Press.

Pask, E (2005) Self-sacrifice, self-transcendence and nurses' professional self. *Nursing Philosophy, 6*(4): 247–254.

Peel, N (2003) Critical care: the role of the critical care nurse in the delivery of bad news. *British Journal of Nursing, 12*: 966–971.

Perrin, EC, Lewkowicz, C and Young, MH (2000) Shared vision: concordance among fathers, mothers, and paediatricians about unmet needs of children with chronic health conditions. *Pediatrics, 105*: 277–285.

Petrie, P (1997) *Communicating with Children and Adults: Interpersonal skills for early years and play work.* London: Arnold.

Pfeffer, J (1981) *Power in Organizations.* Marshfield, MA: Pitman Publishing.

Phillips, A and Taylor, B (2009) *On Kindness.* London: Penguin.

Pinker, S (2011) *The Better Angels of Our Nature: The decline of violence in history and its causes.* London: Penguin.

Plato (344c) (2004) *Plato's Republic.* Indianapolis: Hackett.

Platt, L (2005) *Migration and Social Mobility: The life chances of Britain's minority ethnic communities.* London: Joseph Rowntree Foundation.

Polanyi, M (2009) *The Tacit Dimension.* Chicago: University of Chicago Press.

Popay, J, Whitehead, M and Hunter, D (2010) Injustice is killing people on a large scale – but what is to be done about it? *Journal of Public Health, 32*(2): 148–149.

Porter, S (1991) In: Sweet, S and Norman, I (1995) The nurse–doctor relationship: a selective literature review. *Journal of Advanced Nursing 22*: 165–170.

Potter, J, Hami, F, Bryan, T and Quigley, C (2003) Symptoms in 400 patients referred to palliative services: prevalence and patterns. *Palliative Medicine, 17*: 310–314.

Prilleltensky, I, Nelson, G and Peirson, L (2001) The role of power and control in children's lives: an ecological analysis of pathways towards wellness, resilience and problems. *Journal of Community and Applied Social Psychology, 11*(2): 143–158.

Prosser, J (2013) Judith Butler: queer feminism, transgender, and the transubstantiation of sex. In: Hall, DE, Jagose, A, with Bebell, A and Potter, S (eds). *The Routledge Queer Studies Reader.* London and New York: Routledge.

Quinn, F and Hughes, S (2007) *Quinn's Principles and Practice of Nurse Education*. Oxford: Nelson Thornes.

Radsma, J (1994) Caring and nursing: a dilemma. *Journal of Advanced Nursing, 20*: 444–449.

Rapley, M, Moncrieff, J and Dillon, J (eds). (2011) *De-Medicalizing Misery: Psychiatry, psychology and the human condition*. Basingstoke: Palgrave Macmillan.

Raworth, K (2017) *Doughnut Economics: 7 ways to think like a 21st century economist*. London: Random House, Business Books.

RCN (2012) Going upstream: nursing's contribution to public health. *Prevent, promote and protect*. London: RCN.

Reed, S and Standing, M (2011) *Successful Professional Portfolios for Nursing Students*. Exeter: Learning Matters.

Rees, C and Sheard, C (2004) Undergraduate medical students' views about a reflective portfolio assessment of their communication skills learning. *Medical Education, 38*: 125–128.

Reiger, K and Lane, K (2013) 'How can we go on caring when nobody here cares about us?' Australian public maternity units as contested care sites.(Report). *Women and Birth, 26*(2): 133.

Reynolds, WJ and Scott, B (2000) Do nurses and other professional helpers normally display much empathy? Integrative literature reviews and meta-analyses. *Journal of Advanced Nursing, 31*(1): 226–234.

Richardson, C, Percy, M and Hughes, J (2015) Nursing therapeutics: teaching student nurses care, compassion and empathy. *Nurse Education Today, 35*: e1–e5.

Richardson, L (1997) *Fields of Play (Constructing an Academic Life)*. New Brunswick, NJ: Rutgers University Press.

Riley, AW (2004) Evidence that school-aged children can self-report on their health. *Ambulatory Pediatrics*, 4 (Suppl. 4): 371–376.

Robb, M and Douglas, J (2004) Managing diversity. *Nursing Management UK, 11*(1): 25–29.

Roberts, I and Edwards, P (2010) *The Energy Glut: The politics of fatness in an overheating world*. London: Zed Books.

Roberts, M (2005) The production of the psychiatric subject: power, knowledge and Michel Foucault. *Nursing Philosophy 6*: 33–42.

Rockström, J, Steffen W, Noone, K, et al. (2009) Planetary boundaries: exploring the safe operating space for humanity. *Ecology and Society, 14*(2): 32. Available at: www.ecologyandsociety.org/vol14/iss2/art32/.

Rodgers, BL and Cowles, KV (1997) A conceptual foundation for human suffering in nursing care and research. *Journal of Advanced Nursing, 25*: 1048–1053.

Rogers, CR (1961) *On Becoming a Person*. Boston, MA: Houghton Mifflin.

Rogers, CR (1967) *On Becoming a Person: A therapist's view of psychotherapy.* London: Constable.

Rogers, CR (2002) *Client Centred Therapy.* London: Constable.

Rose, D and Pevalin, DJ (2005) *The National Statistics Socio-Economic Classification: Origins, development and use.* Institute for Social and Economic Research, University of Essex. Basingstoke: Palgrave Macmillan.

Rossiter, A (2007) Chapter 2. In: Mandell, D. *Revisiting the Use of Self: Questioning professional identities.* Toronto: Canadian Scholar's Press.

Ruesch, J (1961) *Therapeutic Communication.* Toronto: Norton.

Ryan, EB and Hamilton, JM (1994) Patronising the old: how do younger and older adults respond to baby talk in the nursing home? *International Journal of Aging and Human Development, 39*(1): 21–32.

Sackett, D, Strauss, S, Richardson, W and Haynes, R (2004) *Evidence Based Medicine: How to practise and teach EBM.* London: Churchill Livingstone.

Sapir, E (1983) In: Mandelbaum, DG (ed.) *Selected Writings of Edward Sapir in Language, Culture and Personality.* Berkeley, CA: University of California Press.

Savage, M, Devine, F, Cunningham, N, et al. (2013) A new model of social class: findings from the BBC's Great British class survey experiment. *Sociology,* April.

Sawley, L (2001) Perceptions of racism in the Health Service. *Nursing Standard, 15*(19): 33–35.

Scambler, G (2012) *The Greedy Bastards Hypothesis.* Available at: https://grahamscambler. wordpress.com/2012/11/04/gbh-greedy-bastards-and-health-inequalities/

Scambler, G (2013a) Resistance in unjust times: Archer, Structured Agency and the Sociology of Health Inequalities. *Sociology, 47*(1): 142–156.

Scambler, G (2013b) *Archer and the Focused Autonomous reflexive.* Available at: www. grahamscambler.com/archer-and-the-focused-autonomous-reflexive/

Schön, D (1987) *Educating the Reflective Practitioner: Toward a new design for teaching and learning in the professions.* San Francisco, CA: Jossey-Bass.

Seddon, J (2008) *Systems Thinking in the Public Sector: The failure of the reform regime … and a manifesto for a better way.* Axminster: Triarchy Press.

Sellman, D (1997) The virtues in the moral education of nurses: Florence Nightingale revisited. *Nursing Ethics, 4*(1): 3–11.

Shields, L, Morrall, P, Goodman, B, Purcell, C and Watson, R (2012) Care to be a nurse? Reflections on a radio broadcast and its ramifications for nursing today. *Nurse Education Today, 32*: 614–617.

Short, NP (2011) Freeze-frame: reflections on being in hospital. In: Grant, A, Biley, F and Walker, H. *Our Encounters with Madness.* Ross-on-Wye: PCCS Books, pp131–138.

Short, N and Grant, A (2016) Poetry as hybrid pedagogy in mental health nurse education. *Nurse Education Today, 43*: 60–63.

Siviter, B and Stevens, D (2004) *The Student Nurse Handbook: A survival guide.* Oxford: Bailliere Tindall.

Sloane, J (1993) Offences and defences against patients: a psychoanalytical view of the borderline between empathic failure and malpractice. *Canadian Journal of Psychology, 38*: 265–273.

Smail, D (2011) Psychotherapy: illusion with no future? In: Rapley, M, Moncrieff, J and Dillon, J (eds). *De-Medicalizing Misery: Psychiatry, psychology and the human condition.* Basingstoke: Palgrave Macmillan, pp226–238.

Smircich, L (1983) Concepts of culture and organizational analysis. *Administrative Science Quarterly, 28*: 339–358.

Smith, A (1997) Learning about reflection. *Journal of Advanced Nursing, 28*: 891–898.

Smith, A and Jack, K (2005) Reflective practice: a meaningful task for students. *Nursing Standard, 19*: 33–37.

Smith, CE (1987) *Patient Education: Nurses in partnership with other health professionals.* Orlando, FL: Grune & Stratton.

Smith, MK (1997, 2004) Eduard Lindeman and the meaning of adult education. In: *The Encyclopaedia of Informal Education.* Available at: www.infed.org/thinkers/et-lind.htm.

Smith, S and Grant, A (2014) Facial affect recognition and mental health. *Mental Health Practice, 17*(10): 12–16.

Smith, S and Grant, A (2016) The corporate construction of psychosis and the rise of the psychosocial paradigm: Emerging implications for mental health nurse education. *Nurse Education Today, 39*: 22–25.

Speed, E (2011) Discourses of acceptance and resistance: speaking out about psychiatry. In: Rapley, M, Moncrieff, J and Dillon, J (eds). *De-Medicalizing Misery: Psychiatry, psychology and the human condition.* Basingstoke: Palgrave Macmillan, pp123–140.

Spicer, A (2017) *Business Bullshit.* London: Routledge.

Spichiger, E, Walhagen, MI and Benner, P (2005) Nursing as a caring practice. *Scandinavian Journal of Caring Science, 19*: 303–309.

Standing, G (2014) *The Precariat: The new dangerous class.* London. Bloomsbury.

Stanley, JC, Hayes, J, Fredrick, L and Silverman, R (2014) Examining student nurses' perceptions of diverse populations: are student nurses prepared to care for culturally diverse patients? *Journal of Nurse Education and Practice, 4*(7): 148–155.

Stein, L (1967) The doctor–nurse game. *Archive of General Psychiatry, 16*: 699–703.

Stein, L, Watts, D and Howell, T (1990) The doctor–nurse game revisited. *New England Journal of Medicine, 322*: 546–549.

Sternberg, RJ (2001) *In Search of the Human Mind,* 3rd edn. Fort Worth, TX: Harcourt College.

Stevens, S (2017) *Five Year Forward View.* Available at: www.england.nhs.uk/wp-content/uploads/2014/10/5yfv-web.pdf.

Stewart, I and Joines, V (2012) TA today. *A New Introduction to Transactional Analysis,* 2nd edn. Melton Mowbray: Lifespace.

Stokes, G (1991) A transcultural nurse is about. *Senior Nurse, 11*(1): 40–42.

Streeck, W (2016) The Post Capitalist Interregnum: the old system is dying but a new social order cannot yet be born. *Juncture, 23*(2): 68–77.

Stuckler, D and Basu, S (2013) *The Body Economic: Why austerity kills.* New York: Basic Books.

Sundin-Huard, D (2001) Subject Positions Theory: its application in understanding collaboration (and confrontation) in critical care. *Journal of Advanced Nursing, 34*(3): 376–382.

Sweeney, A, Clement, S, Filson, B and Kennedy, A (2016) Trauma-informed mental healthcare in the UK: what is it and how can we further its development? *Mental Health Review Journal, 21*(3): 174–192.

Tajfel, H (ed.) (1982) *Social Identity Intergroup Relations.* Cambridge: Cambridge University Press, pp15–40.

Talbot, C (2016) *The Myth of Neoliberalism.* Available at: https://colinrtalbot.wordpress.com/2016/08/31/the-myth-of-neoliberalism/

Tame, S (2012) The effect of continuing professional education on perioperative nurses' relationship with medical staff: findings from a qualitative study. *Journal of Advanced Nursing, 69*(4): 817–827.

Tates, K and Meeuwesen, L (2001) Doctor–parent–child communication: a review of the literature. *Social Science and Medicine, 52:* 839–851.

Taylor, C (2004) *Modern Social Imaginaries.* Chicago: Duke University Press.

Taylor, S, Grant, A and Leigh-Phippard, H (2018) *Our Encounters with Stalking.* Ross on Wye: PCCS Books.

Taylor, S, Leigh-Phippard, H and Grant, A (2014) Writing for recovery: a practice development project for mental health service users, carers and survivors. *International Practice Development Journal, 4*(1): 1–13.

Teekman, B (2000) Exploring reflective practice in nursing. *Journal of Advanced Nursing, 31:* 1125–1135.

The Royal College of Nursing (2017) *#NursingCounts speaking up on nursing pay.* Available at: www.rcn.org.uk/nursingcounts.

Theodosius, C (2008) *Emotional Labour in Health Care: The unmanaged heart of nursing.* London: Routledge.

Thomas, C, Bertram, E, Johnson, D (2009) The SBAR communication technique. *Nurse Educator, 34*(4): 176–180.

Thompson, D (ed.) (1995) *The Concise Oxford Dictionary of Current English,* 9th edn. Oxford: Clarendon Press.

Thompson, N (2001) *Anti-discriminatory Practice,* 3rd edn. Basingstoke: Palgrave Macmillan.

Thorsen, D and Lie, A (2017) *Kva er nyliberalisme? Nyliberalisme – ideer og politisk virkelighet? What is neoliberalism? Neoliberalism ideas and political reality?* Available at: http://folk.uio.no/daget/neoliberalism.pdf.

Thurlow, C (2005) Deconstructing adolescent communication. In: Williams, A and Thurlow, C (eds). *Talking Adolescence: Perspectives on communication in the teenage years.* New York: Peter Lang.

Thwaites, R and Bennett-Levy, J (2007) Conceptualizing empathy in cognitive behaviour therapy: making the implicit explicit. *Behavioural and Cognitive Psychotherapy, 35*: 591–612.

Timmins, F (2007) Communication skills: revisiting the fundamentals. *Nurse Prescribing, 5*: 395–399.

Toffler, A (1980) *The Third Wave.* New York: William Morrow.

Tornstam, L (1997) Gerotranscendence in a Broad Cross Sectional Perspective. *Journal of Aging and Identity, 2*(1): 17–36.

Toynbee, P and Walker, D (2017) *Dismembered: How the attack on the state harms us all.* London: Faber and Faber.

Traynor, M (2014) Caring after Francis: moral failure in nursing reconsidered. *Journal of Research in Nursing, 19*(7–8): 546–556.

Trinder, L and Reynolds, S (eds) (2000) *Evidence-Based Practice: A critical appraisal.* Oxford: Blackwell.

Tuckman, B (1965) Developmental sequence in small groups. *Psychological Bulletin, 63*(6): 384–399.

Turner, JC, Hogg, MA, Oakes, PJ, Reicher, SD and Weatherell, MS (1987) *Rediscovering the Social Group: A social categorisation theory.* Oxford: Blackwell.

United Nations (1989) *United Nations Convention on the Rights of the Child.* Geneva: United Nations.

Walthew, P and Scott, H (2012) Concepts of health promotion held by pre-registration nurses in four schools of nursing in New Zealand. *Nurse Education Today, 32*(3): 224–228.

Watson, J (1988) *Nursing: Human science and human care,* 3rd edn. New York: National League for Nursing.

Watson, J (1997) The theory of human caring: retrospective and prospective. *Nursing Science Quarterly, 10*(1): 49–52.

Watson, J (2015) Jean Watson's Theory of Human Caring. In: Smith, MC and Parker, ME. *Nursing Theories and Nursing Practice,* 4th edn. Philadelphia: F.A. Davis Company, pp321–340.

Watson, J and Foster, R (2003) The attending nurse caring model: integrating theory, evidence and advanced caring-healing therapeutics for transforming professional practice. *Journal of Clinical Nursing, 12*(3): 360–365.

Weedon, C (1987) *Feminist Practice and Poststructuralist Theory.* Oxford: Blackwell.

Whitton, E (2003) *Humanistic Approach to Psychotherapy.* Chichester: Wiley Blackwell.

Whorf, B (1956) In: Carroll, J (ed.) *Language, Thought and Reality: Selected writings of Benjamin Lee Whorf.* Boston, MA: MIT Press.

Wiegratz, J and Whyte, D (2016) *How neoliberalism's moral order feeds fraud and corruption. The Conversation.* Available at: http://theconversation.com/how-neoliberalisms-moral-order-feeds-fraud-and-corruption-60946

Wigens, L and Heathershaw, R (2013) *Mentorship and Clinical Supervision Skills in Health Care,* 2nd edn. Andover: Cengage Learning.

Wilkins, H (1993) Transcultural nursing: a selective review of the literature, 1985–1991. *Journal of Advanced Nursing, 18*: 602–616.

Wilkinson, R and Pickett, K (2009) *The Spirit Level: Why more equal societies almost always do better.* London: Penguin.

Williams, A and Garrett, P (2005) Intergroup perspectives on ageing and intergenerational communication. In: Harwood, J and Giles, H (eds) *Intergroup Communication: Multiple perspectives.* New York: Peter Lang, pp93–115.

Williams, J and Stickley, T (2010) Empathy and nurse education. *Nurse Education Today, 30*: 752–755.

Wittgenstein, L (1972) *Philosophical Investigations.* Oxford: Basil Blackwell.

Wong, L and Gerras, S (2015) *Lying to ourselves: Dishonesty in the army profession.* Carlisle Barracks, PA: Strategic Studies Institute.

World Health Organization (WHO) (2000a) *World Health Report 2000 – Health Systems: Improving performance.* Geneva: WHO.

World Health Organization (WHO) (2000b) *Nurses and Midwives for Health: A WHO strategy for nursing and midwifery education.* Copenhagen: WHO Regional Office for Europe.

World Health Organization Europe (2003) *Nurses and Midwives: A Force for Health.* WHO European Strategy for Continuing Education for Nurses and Midwives. Available at: www.euro.who.int/__data/assets/pdf_file/0016/102238/E81549.pdf.

World Health Organization (2008) *Closing the Gap in a Generation: Health equity through action on the social determinants of health.* Available at: www.who.int/social_determinants/thecommission/finalreport/en/.

Wrate, RM (1992) Talking to adolescents. In: Myerscough, PR (ed.) *Talking with Patients: A basic clinical skill,* 2nd edn. Oxford: Oxford University Press.

Wright, S (2014) Cash v compassion: underpaid care workers expose the battle between the profit and the service ethos, says Stephen Wright. (Reflections). *Nursing Standard, 29* (1): 26.

Wright Mills, C (1959) *The Sociological Imagination.* Oxford: Oxford University Press.

Wu, H and Volker, D (2012) Humanistic theory: application to hospice and palliative care. *Journal of Advanced Nursing, 68*(2): 471–479.

Wurzbach, ME (1999) The moral metaphors of nursing. *Journal of Advanced Nursing, 30*(1): 94–99.

Wyer, RS and Srull, TK (1986) Human cognition in its social context. *Psychological Review, 93*: 322–359.

Young, R, Sweeting, H and West, P (2006) Prevalence of deliberate self harm and attempted suicide within contemporary Goth youth subculture: longitudinal cohort study. *BMJ, 332*(7549): 1058–1061.

Zeeman, L, Aranda, K and Grant, A (2014a) Queer challenges to evidence-based practice. *Nursing Inquiry, 21*(2): 101–111.

Zeeman, L, Aranda, K and Grant, A (eds) (2014b) *Queering Health: Critical challenges to normative health and healthcare.* Ross-on-Wye: PCCS Books.

Zimbardo, P (2009) *The Lucifer Effect.* London: Rider.

Index

Note: References in **bold** are to the Glossary; those to tables and figures are indicated as '69*t*,' '87*f*.'